a LANGE medical book

CURRENT ESSENTIALS
of CRITICAL CARE

Edited by

D1503613

Darryl Y. Sue, MD
Professor of Clinical Medicine
David Geffen School of Medicine at UCLA
Division of Respiratory and Critical Care Physiology and Medicine,
  Department of Medicine,
Harbor-UCLA Medical Center
Torrance, California

Janine R.E. Vintch, MD
Assistant Clinical Professor of Medicine
David Geffen School of Medicine at UCLA
Division of General Internal Medicine and Division of Respiratory and
  Critical Care Physiology and Medicine, Department of Medicine,
Harbor-UCLA Medical Center
Torrance, California

Lange Medical Books/McGraw-Hill
Medical Publishing Division

New York   Chicago   San Francisco   Lisbon   London   Madrid   Mexico City
Milan   New Delhi   San Juan   Seoul   Singapore   Sydney   Toronto

Current Essentials of Critical Care

1 2 3 4 5 6 7 8 9 DOC/DOC 0 1 0 9 8 7 6 5 4

ISBN 0-07-143656-1

ISSN 1550-0705

NOTICE

This book was set in Times Roman by Matrix.
The editors were Jack Farrell, Shelley Reinhardt, Harriet Lebowitz, and Penny Linskey.
The production supervisor was Catherine H. Saggese.
The cover designer was Elizabeth Pisacreta.
The index was prepared by Patricia Perrier.
RR Donnelley was the printer and binder.

This book is printed on acid-free paper.

INTERNATIONAL EDITION ISBN: 0-07-111475-0
Copyright © 2005. Exclusive rights by the McGraw-Hill Companies, Inc., for manufacture and export. This book cannot be re-exported from the country to which it is consigned by McGraw-Hill. The International Edition is not available in North America.

Contents

Contributors

Chan-Chou Chuang, MD
Attending Physician, Division of Respiratory and Critical Care Physiology and Medicine, Department of Medicine, Harbor-UCLA Medical Center
Torrance, California

Brian Korotzer, MD
Assistant Clinical Professor of Medicine, David Geffen School of Medicine at UCLA, Pulmonary and Critical Care Medicine, Kaiser Permanente Medical Center
Bellflower, California

Mark T. Munekata, MD, MPH
Associate Clinical Professor of Medicine, David Geffen School of Medicine at UCLA, Division of General Internal Medicine, Department of Medicine, Harbor-UCLA Medical Center
Torrance, California

Gunter K. Rieg, MD
Assistant Professor of Medicine, David Geffen School of Medicine at UCLA, Division of HIV Medicine, Department of Medicine, Harbor-UCLA Medical Center
Torrance, California

Darryl Y. Sue, MD
Professor of Clinical Medicine, David Geffen School of Medicine at UCLA, Division of Respiratory and Critical Care Physiology and Medicine, Department of Medicine, Harbor-UCLA Medical Center
Torrance, California

Janine R.E. Vintch, MD
Assistant Clinical Professor of Medicine, David Geffen School of Medicine at UCLA, Division of General Internal Medicine and Division of Respiratory and Critical Care Physiology and Medicine, Department of Medicine, Harbor-UCLA Medical Center
Torrance, California

Mallory D. Witt, MD
Associate Professor of Clinical Medicine, David Geffen School of
   Medicine at UCLA, Division of HIV Medicine, Department of
   Medicine, Harbor-UCLA Medical Center
Torrance, California

Preface

Our goal in this book is to provide the reader with only the most crucial and important points for the variety of disorders likely to be encountered in the adult intensive care unit, including the key first steps in diagnosis, confirmation of diagnosis, and initial management strategies. In preparing the manuscript, we were struck by several insights. First was the importance of general supportive care of the patient regardless of the primary diagnosis leading to admission to the ICU. Paying attention to prevention of aspiration pneumonia, reduction of risk for deep venous thrombosis, improving glycemic control, providing nutritional support, and reducing upper gastrointestinal bleeding should be encouraged in all eligible patients. Second, we found that understanding the critically ill patient requires the knowledge and experience of sound training. There can be no substitute for a strong background in basic science (physiology, pharmacology, microbiology, and pathology) combined with training in clinical medicine and skills in the critical analysis of the literature. Finally, we were challenged tremendously in making the decisions about what to include and what to exclude in a book such as this. Thus, while this book gives the reader only the key points, these points focus on what to look for and what to do first in these critically ill patients.

Much of what is done in the ICU has evolved from what seems to be good common sense practice, and only recently has there been evidence-based data supporting how we diagnose and manage critically ill patients. Of course, there remains much to be studied and analyzed, and this reflects how difficult it is to perform valid clinical studies in these unstable and very sick patients. Nevertheless, there is now evidence on adjusting tidal volume in ARDS, controlling glucose in postoperative patients, positioning patients to reduce the risk of nosocomial pneumonia, and preventing complications in status asthmaticus. Those who take care of critically ill patients should look forward to more and better investigations that will help us improve care and outcomes.

Following in the footsteps of *Essentials of Diagnosis and Treatment*, we have tried to include a Clinical Pearl for each topic and to provide one up-to-date reference to guide further reading. Providing these was quite a challenge and we look forward to augmenting and updating both of these features.

We want to thank our colleagues at McGraw-Hill, Jack Farrell, for considering us for this project, and Shelley Reinhardt, for help and encouragement. We are grateful to our contributors for enthusiastically taking on the challenge of this book. Finally, we also would like to thank our families for their support and patience.

Darryl Y. Sue, MD
Janine R.E. Vintch, MD
Torrance, California

Monitoring & Support

Anxiety and Sedation

■ Essentials of Diagnosis
- Distress, often expressed as fear, agitation
- Tachycardia, hypertension, diaphoresis
- May manifest as pain, restlessness, discoordination with mechanical ventilation
- Frequent complaint of patients, sometimes misinterpreted
- Contributing factors include stressful ICU environment, excessive noise, sleep deprivation, painful procedures, mechanical ventilation, medications, anticipation of surgery, fear
- Mechanical ventilation may contribute, especially low tidal volume, permissive hypercapnia

■ Differential Diagnosis
- Hypoxemia
- Alcohol or drug withdrawal
- Hyperthyroidism
- Beta-agonist excess
- Infection, sepsis
- Psychiatric illness, including severe situational reaction to ICU environment

■ Treatment
- Exclude medical conditions, including pain, especially if patient shows delirium
- Explain anticipated events, procedures, current condition to patient; provide orientation to date, time; include family members in discussions, encourage visitation
- Anticipate and control pain; avoid sleep interruptions
- If sedation needed, objective scales for measuring effects of sedation useful; target sedation: follows verbal commands
- For most patients, lorazepam recommended for long-term use; midazolam, propofol useful for short-term sedation

■ Pearl
Daily interruption of sedation reduces duration of mechanical ventilation, length of ICU stay, and number of diagnostic studies for unexplained altered mental status.

Reference

Kress JP et al: Daily interruption of sedative infusions in critically ill patients undergoing mechanical ventilation. N Engl J Med 2000;34:1471. [PMID: 10816184]

Arterial Pressure Monitoring

- **Essential Concepts**
  - Allows continuous, accurate, repeated measurement of blood pressure when needed (hypotension, hypertension, highly vasoactive drugs)
  - Helpful for repeated sampling of arterial blood for blood gases
  - Complications: bleeding, infection, thrombosis, "downstream" arterial emboli with ischemia
  - Contraindications: increased risk of bleeding (coagulopathy, thrombocytopenia), local infection, hypercoagulable states, anticipated use of thrombolytic agents

- **Essentials of Management**
  - Use 16- to 20-g catheter inserted into radial or dorsalis pedis artery
  - Avoid brachial artery (high risk for serious complications) and femoral artery (high risk for bleeding)
  - Attach to continuous pressure infuser with low-dose continuous heparin infusion
  - Measure pressure with transducer attached using nondistensible tubing
  - Remove air bubbles to avoid damped arterial waveform (falsely low systolic and high diastolic pressure)
  - Check insertion site at least daily for bleeding, infection, adequate distal pulses
  - Remove catheter if local complications or within 3–4 days
  - Relative contraindications: coagulopathy or thrombocytopenia, bacteremia, anticipated use of thrombolytic agents
  - Complications during placement: bleeding, arterial damage
  - Complications during use: infection, *in situ* thrombosis, distal arterial emboli with limb ischemia

- **Pearl**

Arterial catheter blood pressure may be lower or higher than measured by cuff, depending on vascular disease, age, and stroke volume.

Reference

Martin C et al: Long-term arterial cannulation in ICU patients using the radial artery or dorsalis pedis artery. Chest 2001;119:901. [PMID: 11243975]

Central Venous Pressure Monitoring

- ■ Essential Concepts
  - Pressure in central vein measured by catheter placed near entrance to right atrium
  - Reflects filling pressure or preload to right ventricle
  - Normal central venous pressure (CVP) -4 to 10 mm Hg
  - Lower in patients with low intravascular volume
  - Higher CVP may mean volume overload, right ventricular failure (chronic: cor pulmonale; acute: right ventricular infarction), especially if CVP $>$ pulmonary artery wedge pressure, or pericardial effusion/cardiac tamponade
  - Use CVP to estimate volume status; but inaccurate in pulmonary hypertension, respiratory failure, right heart failure

- ■ Essentials of Management
  - Insert central venous catheter via internal jugular or subclavian vein using sterile technique
  - Measure CVP using water manometer (1.36 cm H_2O = 1 mm Hg) or strain gauge pressure transducer (electronic measurement) at end-expiration
  - Volume depletion suggested by CVP $<$ 5 mm Hg or especially by initial increase followed by rapid fall in CVP after intravenous volume challenge (250–500 mL)
  - For adequate volume challenge, use target CVP 8–12 mm Hg
  - Complications: bleeding, pneumothorax, catheter infection, thrombosis, pulmonary thromboembolism, air embolism (rarely)

- ■ Pearl

Measure O_2 saturation from blood drawn from central venous catheter. Low values may indicate inadequate systemic perfusion, similar to "mixed venous blood" drawn from pulmonary artery catheter.

Reference

McGee DC et al: Preventing complications of central venous catheterization. N Engl J Med 2003;348:1123. [PMID: 12646670]

Deep Venous Thrombosis, Prevention in Medical Patients

- **Essential Concepts**
  - High deep venous thrombosis (DVT) and pulmonary embolism (PE) risk in surgical or medical patients (15–50%); with myocardial infarction (24%), strokes
  - Risk increased by stasis, immobilization, release of thromboplastins, hypercoagulable state (transient or chronic), infection, local venous trauma
  - Preventive therapy indicated for all patients in ICU, unless contraindicated
  - Intensity of treatment depends on underlying disease or procedure, risk of DVT, and likelihood of early ambulation

- **Essentials of Management**
  - LDUH = subcutaneous low-dose heparin, 5000–7000 units, 2–3 times daily; LMWH = subcutaneous low molecular weight heparin; ES = elastic stockings; SCD = sequential compression device
  - Acute myocardial infarction: LDUH or IV heparin (aPTT 46–70 s)
  - Ischemic stroke with impaired mobility: LDUH or LMWH; if anticoagulation contraindicated, ES or SCD
  - Medical illness without contraindication: LDUH or LMWH plus ES or SCD; if contraindication, ES plus SCD

- **Pearl**

Even patients with hemorrhagic strokes should be considered for DVT prophylaxis, but they should be closely observed to determine if the stroke is extending.

Reference

Geerts WH et al: Prevention of venous thromboembolism. Chest 2001;119(1 Suppl):132S. [PMID: 11157647]

Deep Venous Thrombobosis, Prevention in Surgical Patients

- **Essential Concepts**
  - Highest deep venous thrombosis (DVT) and pulmonary embolism (PE) risk after hip fracture, total hip or knee replacement (40–70%); postoperative surgery patients (25%)

- **Essentials of Management**
  - LDUH = subcutaneous low-dose heparin, 5000–7000 units, 2–3 times daily; LMWH = subcutaneous low molecular weight heparin; ES = elastic stockings; SCD = sequential compression device; ADW = adjusted-dose warfarin
  - General surgery, low risk (age < 40; minor procedure): early ambulation; moderate risk (minor procedure with risk factors; minor surgery age 40–60, no risks; major surgery age < 40, no risks): LDUH, LMWH, ES, or SCD
  - General surgery: high risk with bleeding likely: ES or SCD; very high risk for DVT: LDUH or LMWH plus ES or SCD
  - Gynecologic surgery, major, benign: LDUH twice/daily; or LMWH or SCD before and after surgery; extensive, malignant: LDUH three times/day plus ES or SCD; or higher dose LMWH
  - Urologic surgery, brief, minor: early ambulation; major open: LMWH, LDUH, ES, or SCD; highest-risk: LDUH or LMWH plus ES with or without SCD
  - Total hip replacement: LMWH (12 hours before or 12 to 24 hours after; or half usual high-risk dose 4 to 6 hours after, usual high-risk dose following day); or ADW therapy (INR 2.5), started pre- or immediately postoperatively
  - Total knee replacement: LMWH or ADW (INR 2.5); alternative, optimal use of SCD
  - Hip-fracture surgery: LMWH or ADW (INR 2.5)
  - Intracranial neurosurgery: SCD with or without ES; LDUH or postoperative LMWH
  - Head trauma, thrombosis risk: LMWH as soon as safe; if delayed or contraindicated, ES and SCD; if suboptimal prophylaxis, look for DVT; IVC filter if found
  - Acute spinal cord injury: LMWH plus ES and SCD; if contraindicated, ES and SCD

- **Pearl**

Epidural or spinal anesthesia in anticoagulated patients may cause paraspinous hematomas, which can lead to long-term neurological deficits.

Reference

Geerts WH et al: Prevention of venous thromboembolism. Chest 2001;119(1 Suppl):132S. [PMID: 11157647]

Delirium

■ Essentials of Diagnosis

- Agitation, altered sensorium, disorientation, waxing and waning of level of consciousness, incoherent speech
- Common problem, especially with advanced age, neuropsychiatric disorders, alcoholism, drug overdose, use of multiple medications, anemia; less common: chemical exposure, hepatic encephalopathy, hypoxemia, cerebral hypoperfusion, hyponatremia, hypercalcemia, renal failure
- Medications (neuroleptics, corticosteroids, lidocaine, cimetidine, antihistamines, benzodiazepines); withdrawal from alcohol or sedative-hypnotic drugs
- ICU environment contributes to sleep deprivation, disorientation, stress, but is almost never the only cause
- Delirium prolongs ICU stay, contributes to morbidity and mortality

■ Differential Diagnosis

- Anxiety, depression, psychosis; treatment with neuroleptic agents, neuroleptic malignant syndrome

■ Treatment

- Assess for hypoxemia, hypotension, fluid and electrolyte problems, sepsis, meningitis, stroke, intracranial hemorrhage, withdrawal from alcohol or sedative-hypnotic drugs
- Review medications, blood count, serum electrolytes, arterial blood gases
- Protect from falls, disconnection of life support (endotracheal tube, intravenous catheters); orient to location and time
- Consider benzodiazepines (lorazepam), haloperidol, or combination, if needed
- Complications of treatment: oversedation, respiratory depression, hypotension; for haloperidol–prolonged QT interval, dystonic reactions, rarely neuroleptic malignant syndrome

■ Pearl

Delirium from withdrawal from alcohol or benzodiazepines may begin as late as 5–7 days after stopping consumption.

Reference

McNicoll L et al: Delirium in the intensive care unit: occurrence and clinical course in older patients. J Am Geriatr Soc 2003;5:591. [PMID: 12752832]

Depression

- **Essentials of Diagnosis**
  - Complaints of unhappiness, worthlessness, hopelessness, lack of planning for future, guilt; but anticipate depressed mood in all ICU patients regardless of symptoms
  - Decreased interest in condition, treatment plans, physical and mental activities; may exhibit lack of cooperation, refusal to agree to treatment or discuss with family
  - Suicidal ideation, lack of self-esteem
  - 10–40% of seriously ill, hospitalized patients have depression; but only 25–33% are diagnosed
  - May be related to underlying major psychiatric illness

- **Differential Diagnosis**
  - Medications: beta-blockers, sedatives, antihypertensives
  - Endocrinopathies: hypothyroidism, hyperadrenalism
  - Hyponatremia, hypoxia
  - Major depression
  - Sleep deprivation
  - Alcohol or substance abuse or withdrawal

- **Treatment**
  - Maximize interactions with family, visitors, nursing and physician staff; include patients in decision-making, daily activities; provide realistic support and prognostic information
  - Improve sleep quantity and quality
  - Anxiolytic agents may be helpful
  - Consider psychiatric consultation, if severe, or pharmacologic antidepressant therapy planned
  - Antidepressant drugs limited by side effects in critically ill patients; selective serotonin reuptake inhibitors (SSRIs) less hazardous than tricyclic antidepressants; start SSRIs at low dose, gradual titration upwards, such as paroxetine 5–10 mg, sertraline 12.5–25 mg, fluoxetine 5 mg; effect may take days

- **Pearl**

A depressed mood in seriously ill hospitalized adults is independently associated with increased mortality, after adjustment for disease severity and functional status.

Reference

Roach MJ et al: Depressed mood and survival in seriously ill hospitalized adults. The SUPPORT Investigators. Arch Intern Med 1998;158:397. [PMID: 9487237]

End-Tidal P_{CO_2} Monitoring

- **Essential Concepts**
  - In spontaneously breathing normal patients, end-tidal P_{CO_2} (P_{ETCO_2}) approximates arterial P_{CO_2} (Pa_{CO_2})
  - Difference between P_{ETCO_2} and Pa_{CO_2} widens in patients with lung disease (pneumonia, asthma, COPD, ARDS, pulmonary embolism)
  - Increased Pa_{CO_2}–P_{ETCO_2} difference associated with high dead-space/tidal volume ratio (V_D/V_T)
  - Unpredictable Pa_{CO_2} − P_{ETCO_2} differences with irregular breathing, tachypnea, prolonged exhalation
  - P_{ETCO_2} cannot be substituted for Pa_{CO_2} when making ventilator changes or determining hyper- or hypoventilation
  - Capnography looks at expiratory CO_2 concentration continuously; may be useful for estimating endotracheal tube cuff leak

- **Essentials of Management**
  - Measure arterial P_{CO_2} to determine Pa_{CO_2} − P_{ETCO_2} difference
  - Normal Pa_{CO_2} − P_{ETCO_2} = −2 to 0 mm Hg
  - Use P_{ETCO_2} to confirm endotracheal tube placement
  - High Pa_{CO_2} − P_{ETCO_2} difference predicts high V_D/V_T, potential difficulty with weaning
  - If Pa_{CO_2} − P_{ETCO_2} difference remains constant (only rarely), changes in P_{ETCO_2} may be used for adjusting minute ventilation.
  - Increased Pa_{CO_2} − P_{ETCO_2} difference may be sign of pulmonary embolism
  - Attach CO_2 monitoring probe to end of endotracheal or tracheostomy tube according to directions

- **Pearl**

P_{ETCO_2} reflects perfusion of the lungs, which is related to cardiac output, much more than the arterial P_{CO_2}, which reflects ventilation.

Reference

Anderson CT et al: Carbon dioxide kinetics and capnography during critical care. Crit Care 2000; 4:207 [PMID: 11094503]

Geriatric Patient Considerations

- **Essential Concepts**
  - Decline in maximum functional capacity of all organ systems with aging; normally functioning elderly have less reserve
  - Normal arterial PaO_2, creatinine clearance, VC, FEV_1 decline with age
  - Drug metabolism and clearance reduced in older adults
  - Delirium common in older patients in ICU, especially with cognitive impairment, fractures, neuroleptic drugs, infection, opioids
  - Manifestations of disease more subtle, unusual; may be lack of fever with infection
  - Have lower proportion of total body water (45–50%); lower lean body mass/muscle mass
  - More prone to DVT, decubitus ulcers, malnutrition, insufficient fluid intake, falls, fractures, renal insufficiency, inadvertent drug interactions or overdosage, delirium, muscle atrophy
  - Outcome of severe illness worse in elderly; higher mortality from sepsis, ARDS, acute renal failure, respiratory failure

- **Essentials of Management**
  - Adjust medications for expected decreases in renal, liver function; extra caution with digoxin, beta-blockers, ACE inhibitors, nephrotoxic antibiotics, radiographic contrast
  - Expect more subtle and milder findings, even in severe illness
  - Limit use of sedatives, opiates, antihistamines, neuroleptic drugs unless necessary
  - Avoid sleep disruption, orient patient frequently, provide reassurance, minimal use of restraints
  - Encourage visitors, family participation in care

- **Pearl**

Elderly patients often are prescribed many different drugs ("polypharmacy"); the risk of an adverse drug reaction increases exponentially when four or more drugs are being given.

Reference

Bo M et al: Predictive factors of in-hospital mortality in older patients admitted to a medical intensive care unit. J Am Geriatr Soc 2003;51:529. [PMID: 12657074]

Hyperglycemia, Management in the ICU

- **Essential Concepts**
  - Elevated blood glucose
  - Hyperglycemia affects fluid balance, possibly alters white blood cell function, impairs complement activity
  - Increases mortality following stroke and myocardial infarction
  - Demonstrated benefits of tight glycemic control: decreased wound infection following coronary artery bypass surgery; decreased mortality in diabetics following myocardial infarction; decreased mortality, bacteremia, critical illness polyneuropathy in patients admitted to surgical ICU
  - Differential diagnosis: diabetes mellitus, laboratory error, stress, steroid induced diabetes

- **Essentials of Management**
  - Initiate intravenous infusion of insulin: titrate to goal blood glucose of 80 to 120 mg/dL; use of insulin infusion protocol helpful
  - Consider switching to subcutaneous injections of long-acting insulin once at stable regimen
  - Monitor for and attempt to avoid hypoglycemia

- **Pearl**

Intensive insulin therapy to treat hyperglycemia in critically ill patients, which may be due to illness related insulin resistance and not to previously known diabetes, appears to improve morbidity and mortality.

Reference

Montori VM et al: Hyperglycemia in acutely ill patients. JAMA 2002;288:2167. [PMID: 12413377]

Intracranial Pressure Monitoring

- **Essential Concepts**
  - Intracranial compartment in adults has fixed volume due to rigid skull; contains brain, cerebrospinal fluid (CSF), cerebral blood volume; increase in size of any one of these can lead to elevation of intracranial pressure (ICP)
  - ICP measurements can estimate cerebral perfusion pressure (CPP): CPP = MAP − ICP where MAP is mean arterial pressure; CPP at or above 70 mm Hg by increasing MAP or decreasing ICP may improve survival
  - ICP monitoring techniques used in management of severe head injury, subarachnoid hemorrhage, Reye syndrome, hepatic encephalopathy, other disorders causing intracranial hypertension
  - Controlling ICP in < 20 mm Hg range associated with improved outcome
  - Increased morbidity and mortality associated with ICP > 20 mm Hg that persists for more than 10 to 15 minutes, particularly in patients with severe closed head injuries

- **Essentials of Management**
  - Several monitoring systems available: catheters, hollow screw or bolt, fiberoptic transducer tipped catheters
  - Devices can be placed into several locations: lateral ventricle, intraparenchymal, subdural or subarachnoid space, epidural space
  - Intraventricular catheters remain gold standard in most cases with added benefit of CSF drainage to help control elevated pressures
  - Complications include hemorrhage, hematoma formation, infection, cortical damage

- **Pearl**

Misinterpretation of the data obtained from an ICP monitoring system may result in improper choice of therapeutic intervention.

Reference

Doyle DJ et al: Analysis of intracranial pressure. J Clin Monit 1992;8:81. [PMID: 1538258]

Nutrition, Enteral

- **Essential Concepts**
  - Enteral feeding preferred over parenteral; better outcome, fewer infections, maintenance of GI function
  - Enteral formulas supply calories and protein, vitamins, trace elements
  - Most contain protein hydrolysates, simple and complex carbohydrates, medium chain triglycerides; others elemental (amino acids, sugars)
  - Enteral nutrition formulary includes standard formula (1 cal/mL); formulas for fluid restriction, higher or lower protein, hepatic encephalopathy (high branch chain amino acids)
  - Use nasogastric tubes designed for enteral feeding or gastrostomy or jejunostomy tubes

- **Essentials of Management**
  - Start enteral feeding support in all patients who have no contraindication; no indication for parenteral feeding
  - Determine nutritional status and requirements
  - Select enteral feeding formula based on underlying diseases, patient's volume status, protein and calorie requirements
  - Choose starting and goal target rate (generally 60–90 mL/h for continuous feeding); use enteral feeding pump
  - Place and check position of nasogastric or gastrostomy tube; elevate head of bed 30–45 degrees during feeding to avoid aspiration pneumonia
  - In cases of malnutrition, hypoalbuminemia, diarrhea or prolonged disuse of GI tract, begin feeding at low rate and advance over 24 hours to goal.
  - Consider metoclopramide or erythromycin (promotility agents) if high gastric residual volume
  - Complications: high gastric residual volume (check every 2–4 hours), diarrhea, abdominal distension, aspiration pneumonia

- **Pearl**

If diarrhea persists after slowing feeding rate and diluting formula with sterile water, consider antibiotic-induced diarrhea or C difficile infection.

Reference

ASPEN Board of Directors and the Clinical Guidelines Task Force. Guidelines for the use of parenteral and enteral nutrition in adult and pediatric patients. JPEN J Parenter Enteral Nutr 2002;26(1 Suppl):1SA. [PMID: 11841046]

Nutrition, Parenteral

- ■ Essential Concepts
  - • Enteral feeding superior to parenteral nutrition; parenteral indicated only if patient unable to be fed enterally
  - • Supplies intravenous calories and protein, vitamins, trace elements from amino acids, high concentrations of dextrose, and lipid emulsions (as mixture or separately)
  - • Hospitals have standard formula (20–25% dextrose plus 3–5% amino acids); formulas for fluid restriction, high or restricted protein, hepatic encephalopathy (high branch chain/low aromatic amino acids)
  - • Total parenteral nutrition (TPN) meets caloric and protein needs of critically ill; administered through a central vein
  - • Peripheral parenteral nutrition (PPN): limited calories and protein through peripheral veins; will generally not meet needs of critically ill
  - • Specific indications: short bowel syndrome, high output GI fistula, hyperemesis gravidarum, nonfunctional gut with severe hypoalbuminemia

- ■ Essentials of Management
  - • Determine nutritional status and requirements
  - • Select parenteral nutrition formula based on underlying disease, fluid volume status, protein and calorie requirement
  - • Add insulin (1–5 units/h) to maintain blood glucose < 110 mg/100 mL; adjust electrolytes (Na, K, Cl, acetate); check electrolytes daily; glucose every 4 hours initially, then daily; if giving lipid emulsions, check serum triglycerides daily at start
  - • Complications: fluid overload, hyperglycemia, hypokalemia, hypophosphatemia, sepsis, hyperlipidemia, insertion site infection, candidemia, abnormal liver function tests, metabolic acidosis

- ■ Pearl

Hepatic steatosis, intrahepatic cholestasis and biliary sludge associated with total parenteral nutrition can be prevented, if possible, by concomitant enteral feeding.

Reference

ASPEN Board of Directors and the Clinical Guidelines Task Force. Guidelines for the use of parenteral and enteral nutrition in adult and pediatric patients. JPEN J Parenter Enteral Nutr 2002;26(1 Suppl):1SA. [PMID: 11841046]

Nutritional Support

- **Essential Concepts**
  - Critically ill patients often malnourished beforehand; severe illness associated with increased breakdown of lean body mass (catabolism) due to inflammatory response and high caloric requirements
  - Increase catabolic rate highest in burns, head injury, sepsis, postsurgery, trauma
  - Nutritional support may minimize loss of body stores of energy and protein; inadequate support increases infection, organ failure, mechanical ventilator dependence, mortality, length of hospitalization

- **Essentials of Management**
  - Nutritional support for all patients in ICU, but especially after 3–5 days without nutrition
  - Consult dietitian to estimate calorie and protein needs
  - Low serum albumin indicates poor nutritional status, correlates with outcome
  - For adults, estimate 30–35 kcal/kg ideal body weight plus 1.2–1.5 g protein per kg ideal body weight to start
  - Ideal weight (kg): adult men = 50 + 2.7 kg/inch for heights over 60 inches; adult women = 45.5 + 2.3 kg/inch for heights over 60 inches
  - Higher calorie needs for febrile or septic patients; higher protein needs for burns, head injury; reduce protein intake with acute renal failure (nondialyzed), hepatic encephalopathy
  - Begin support as soon as possible, except with contraindications (lack of access, intolerant of fluids, unable to position properly)
  - Enteral feeding preferred over parenteral nutrition
  - Follow serum electrolytes, albumin, prealbumin, urine urea nitrogen

- **Pearl**

The most accurate measurements of nutritional requirements are made using indirect calorimetry (from oxygen uptake) and nitrogen balance (protein), but these are not shown to improve patient outcome.

Reference

ASPEN Board of Directors and the Clinical Guidelines Task Force. Guidelines for the use of parenteral and enteral nutrition in adult and pediatric patients. JPEN J Parenter Enteral Nutr 2002;26(1 Suppl):1SA. [PMID: 11841046]

Obesity, Severe

- **Essential Concepts**
  - Severe obesity (body mass index [BMI]) > 28) may be associated with increased ICU mortality and complications
  - Linked directly to obesity-hypoventilation syndrome (OHS), obstructive sleep apnea (OSA), restrictive lung disease
  - Risk factor for malignancy, heart failure, coronary artery disease, hypertension, diabetes mellitus, glucose intolerance, respiratory failure, deep venous thrombosis, pulmonary embolism, nonalcoholic steatohepatitis, decubitus ulcers, hip fractures
  - Jeopardizes weaning from mechanical ventilation because of increased breathing work
  - Complicates mechanical ventilator settings, drug dosing, nutritional support calculations, fluid and electrolyte replacement
  - Total body water as proportion of weight falls in obesity (35–40%) compared to 50–60% in nonobese
  - Extremely obese unable to have CT imaging, cardiac catheterization, angiography

- **Essentials of Management**
  - Calculate most drug dosages for "ideal weight" estimated from height, not actual weight in obese
  - Dosage of low molecular weight heparin unreliable in obesity
  - Use ideal weight estimated from height for setting tidal volume during mechanical ventilation; eg, 6 mL/kg ideal body weight High peak and plateau airway pressures due to non-compliant chest wall (diaphragm) do not increase risk of barotrauma
  - Most obese patients have normal to low lean body mass; nutritional support important to maintain function; estimate calorie, protein, fluid needs from ideal weight

- **Pearl**

To estimate "ideal" weight in kg: adult men = 50 + 2.7 kg/inch over 60 inches tall; adult women = 45.5 + 2.3 kg /inch over 60 inches tall.

Reference

El-Solh A et al: Morbid obesity in the medical ICU. Chest 2000; 120:1989. [PMID: 11742933]

Pain

- **Essentials of Diagnosis**
  - Frequent complaint of ICU patients; relief of pain results in better outcomes
  - May not be expressed by patient, especially if sedated, delirious, altered level of consciousness; may show restlessness, confusion, agitation
  - Tachycardia, hypertension, diaphoresis; may increase oxygen consumption, myocardial oxygen demand
  - Anxiety increases pain response
  - Adequate analgesia sometimes avoided for fear of respiratory depression, hypotension, alteration of sensorium, ileus

- **Differential Diagnosis**
  - Hypoxemia
  - Drug reactions
  - Anxiety
  - Delirium

- **Treatment**
  - Anticipate and treat pain from procedures, mechanical ventilation, postsurgery
  - Use objective pain scales to evaluate and adjust analgesia; titrate analgesics to desired effect
  - Explain potentially painful procedures in advance
  - Morphine sulfate preferred analgesia for pain in critically ill
  - Fentanyl preferred if hemodynamically unstable, histamine release with morphine, morphine allergy
  - Consider patient-controlled analgesia in selected patients
  - Anxiolytics, sedation (benzodiazepines) useful adjuncts, not substitutes for adequate analgesia

- **Pearl**

Avoid meperidine in critically ill patients; metabolites cause neuroexcitability and have adverse drug interactions.

Reference

Jacobi J et al: Clinical practice guidelines for the sustained use of sedatives and analgesics in the critically ill adult. Crit Care Med 2002;30:119. [PMID: 11902253]

Pulmonary Artery Catheter

- ■ Essential Concepts
  - • Measures pressure in pulmonary artery (PA), central venous pressure (CVP), and pulmonary artery wedge pressure (PAWP) (estimate of left atrial pressure)
  - • Most measure cardiac output using thermodilution; some with oximeter probe for mixed venous O_2 saturation
  - • Blood can be sampled from distal tip (mixed venous blood) or from proximal port (central venous blood)
  - • Calculate cardiac index (CI), systemic vascular resistance (SVR), and pulmonary vascular resistance (PVR)

- ■ Essentials of Management
  - • Indications: cardiogenic shock, cardiogenic pulmonary edema, acute myocardial infarction with hemodynamic compromise, cardiac tamponade
  - • May be helpful in patients with acute hypoxemic respiratory failure, sepsis and septic shock, but value unknown
  - • Use caution in estimating PAWP with tachycardia, pulmonary hypertension, large intrathoracic pressure swings during respiratory cycle
  - • Measure pressures at "end-expiration"
  - • Inflate balloon only enough to achieve "wedge" position (do not exceed 1.5 mL)
  - • Optimal PAWP = 18 mm Hg in patient with cardiogenic shock
  - • Increased pulmonary edema (normal lungs) when PAWP > 25 mm Hg; in noncardiogenic pulmonary edema, PAWP should be < 10 mm Hg, if patient is hemodynamically stable
  - • Mixed venous P_{O_2} < 30 mm Hg associated with poor organ oxygenation and lactic acidosis; but > 30 mm Hg is not a reliable sign of adequate oxygenation
  - • Relative contraindications: coagulopathy, thrombocytopenia, bacteremia, anticipated use of thrombolytic agents
  - • Complications: bleeding, pneumothorax, arrhythmias, heart block and bradycardia, pulmonary artery, infection

- ■ Pearl

In cardiac tamponade, look for equalization of RA and LA pressures by displaying pressure waveforms on same screen at same scale.

Reference
Cruz K, Franklin C: The pulmonary artery catheter: uses and controversies. Crit Care Clin 2001;17:271-91. [PMID: 11450316]

Pulse Oximetry

- **Essential Concepts**
  - Finger, ear, or other cutaneous probe measures transmission or reflectance of red and infrared light through tissue
  - Pulsatile absorbance ("beat-to-beat") determines percentage of oxyhemoglobin in blood
  - Oxyhemoglobin, carboxyhemoglobin, and methemoglobin read as "oxyhemoglobin"
  - Pulsatile waveform essential for calculation; low perfusion, hypotension, arterial disease, motion artifacts interfere with measurement
  - Correlates well with arterial blood O_2 saturation

- **Essentials of Management**
  - Use for routine monitoring of patients in ICU and during endoscopy, bronchoscopy, minor surgery, suctioning, sleep apnea episodes, bronchodilator therapy
  - Use to adjust supplemental oxygen therapy, including mechanical ventilation
  - Provides estimate of arterial oxygenation; still need arterial blood gases for $Paco_2$ and pH.
  - Do not use to exclude significant carboxyhemoglobinemia (eg, after smoke inhalation)
  - May not be accurate during cardiopulmonary resuscitation
  - Attach to ear lobe or finger according to manufacturer's instructions
  - Check for pulsatile waveform on monitor (if provided)
  - If waveform is poor or pulse oximeter does not provide an adequate reading, try other locations

- **Pearl**

Very high methemoglobin levels have the peculiar effect of causing the pulse oximeter to read 75% regardless of concentration or oxygenation.

Reference

Lee WW et al: The accuracy of pulse oximetry in the emergency department. Am J Emerg Med 2000;18:427. [PMID: 10919532]

Upper GI Bleeding, Prevention

- Essential Concepts
  - 10–25% incidence of shallow, stress-induced ulceration of gastric mucosa with subclinical or clinically important upper GI bleeding in critically ill patients; associated with poor outcome, increased mortality
  - May have clinical bleeding or persistent unexplained fall in hemoglobin
  - Risk factors: mechanical ventilation, coagulopathy, thrombocytopenia, renal failure, burns, postsurgical, possibly lack of enteral feeding, aspirin; may be due to cytokine-mediated decrease in upper GI mucosal resistance to gastric acid, *H pylori*, multiorgan system failure, impaired hemostasis, medications, decreased mucosal blood flow

- Essentials of Management
  - Give prophylactic therapy for all patients receiving mechanical ventilation, with thrombocytopenia, qualitative platelet dysfunction, coagulopathy, significant burns, renal or liver failure
  - Consider in all patients in ICU, especially if hypotension, low cardiac output, inability to feed enterally
  - Sucralfate, a nonantacid, possibly associated with less nosocomial pneumonia; may be less effective
  - For antacid therapies, best results with pH > 4.0 (measurement of pH not clinically indicated)
  - Ranitidine, 150 mg IV per day, continuous infusion or every 8 hours, or famotidine 20 mg IV every 12 hours; adjust for renal insufficiency.
  - Alternative: pantoprazole 40 mg IV daily for 5–7 days, then switch to oral pantoprazole or omeprazole

- Pearl

Patients with highest risk for stress-related upper GI bleeding are those receiving mechanical ventilation and those with disorders tending to lead to bleeding.

Reference

Steinberg KP: Stress-related mucosal disease in the critically ill patient: risk factors and strategies to prevent stress-related bleeding in the intensive care unit. Crit Care Med 2002;30(6 Suppl):S362. [PMID: 1207266]

2

ICU Supportive Care for Specific Medical Problems

Burn Patients

■ **Essential Concepts**

- Assess burn depth: first-degree burns red, dry, painful; second-degree burns red, wet, very painful; third-degree burns leathery, dry, insensate
- Assess extent of total body surface area (TBSA) involved: in adults each body segment assigned 9%: head and neck; anterior chest; posterior chest; anterior abdomen; posterior abdomen including buttocks; each upper extremity; each thigh; each leg and foot; genitals assigned 1%
- Attention to surrounding circumstances important to identify potential toxic exposures; evaluate for associated injuries: neurologic and musculoskeletal examinations
- Patients sustaining serious burns should be transferred to burn center based on American Burn Association criteria: any burn > 10% TBSA in patients < 10 or > 50 years of age; burns involving > 20% TBSA; second- and third-degree burns involving face, hands, feet, genitalia, perineum, major joints; third-degree burns > 5% TBSA; significant electrical, chemical, inhalational burns

■ **Essentials of Management**

- Maintenance of cardiopulmonary function including intubation and mechanical ventilation if airway compromised or breathing appears insufficient
- Immediate fluid resuscitation with half estimated needs administered within first 8 hours; use formulas based on body size, depth, extent of burn to estimate fluid needs; most recommend avoiding colloid during first 24 hours and using crystalloid solutions
- Escharotomy may be necessary to prevent secondary ischemic tissue necrosis and to relieve elevated tissue pressures
- Topical antimicrobial therapy with mafenide, silver sulfadiazine, silver nitrate may decrease incidence of invasive infection
- Increased metabolic rates in postburn period increase caloric and protein needs; require early nutritional support

■ **Pearl**

Burns involving more than 25% of the total body surface area require intravenous fluid resuscitation because ileus precludes oral resuscitation.

Reference

Sheridan RL: Burns. Crit Care Med 2002 Nov;30:S500. [PMID: 12528792]

Chronic Renal Failure Patients

- **Essential Concepts**
  - Elevated BUN and creatinine present over weeks to years
  - Malaise, nausea, hiccups, pruritis, confusion, metallic taste, impotence
  - Hypertension, fluid overload, uremic fetor, pericardial friction rub, asterixis, sallow complexion
  - Anemia, platelet dysfunction, metabolic acidosis, hyperkalemia
  - Hyperphosphatemia and hypocalcemia lead to renal osteodystrophy
  - Renal imaging reveals bilateral small echogenic kidneys

- **Essentials of Management**
  - Renal biopsy not helpful in identifying underlying cause
  - Sodium and fluid restriction; blood pressure control
  - Nutritional support: protein restriction (unless receiving hemodialysis), reduced dietary potassium and phosphorus
  - Avoid hypotension, excessive diuresis
  - Avoid nephrotoxic agents: aminoglycosides, NSAIDs, contrast agents
  - Monitor medications interfering with creatinine clearance: ACE inhibitors, histamine blockers, trimethoprim
  - Adjust dosages of medications eliminated by kidneys
  - Avoid excessive magnesium-containing compounds: antacids, laxatives
  - Administer oral phosphate binders
  - Correct metabolic acidosis, especially if limited ventilatory capacity
  - Recombinant erythropoietin with or without iron for anemia
  - Monitor for cardiac tamponade when pericarditis present
  - Urgent hemodialysis if severe acidosis, hyperkalemia with ECG changes, fluid overload, symptomatic uremia
  - Kidney transplantation

- **Pearl**

While severe hypocalcemia is a common laboratory finding in chronic renal failure, clinical manifestations of tetany are rarely seen because ionized calcium is favorably increased in the setting of acidemia that accompanies chronic renal impairment.

Reference

Yu HT: Progression of chronic renal failure. Arch Intern Med 2003;163:1417. [PMID: 12824091]

Pregnant Patients

- **Essential Concepts**
  - Altered maternal physiology, presence of fetus, diseases specific to pregnancy make management challenging
  - Organ systems adapt to optimize fetal and maternal outcome
  - Cardiovascular system: electrical axis changes with lateral deviation of apex; cardiac output, heart rate, stroke volume increase; reduced peripheral vascular resistance leads to decreased systemic blood pressure
  - Respiratory system: minute ventilation increases in excess of need for oxygen delivery; "hyperventilation of pregnancy" hormonally mediated and results in decreased $Paco_2$ (28 to 32 mm Hg); compensatory bicarbonate loss maintains normal pH
  - Hematologic system: disproportionate plasma volume increase compared to red cell mass leads to "dilutional anemia"; increased thromboembolic risk due to alterations in clotting factors, venous stasis, vessel wall injury
  - Laboratory changes: creatinine decreases while creatinine clearance increases; elevated alkaline phosphatase related to placental production

- **Essentials of Management**
  - Position: avoid supine position after 20 weeks gestation; right lateral decubitus or Fowler position (head of bed elevated) preferred for immobilized patient
  - Monitoring: fetal heart tones should be part of vital signs; continuous fetal monitoring after 23 weeks' gestation if maternal condition affects cardiopulmonary function
  - Thromboembolism prophylaxis: unfractionated or low molecular weight heparin if not contraindicated; venous compression stockings of lesser benefit
  - Nutrition: address early as pregnant women more susceptible to starvation ketosis
  - Imaging studies: ionizing radiation known to be teratogenic; limit radiographs appropriately but do not withhold if results may lead to therapeutic intervention

- **Pearl**

Although care of the mother is the primary concern in most circumstances, attention must also be paid to fetal health and well-being.

Reference

Naylor DF et al: Critical care obstetrics and gynecology. Crit Care Clin 2003;19:127. [PMID: 12688581]

Solid Organ Transplant Recipients

- **Essential Concepts**
  - High risk for complications related to transplanted organ, anatomical disturbances, immunosuppressive therapies
  - Graft failure and chronic rejection major concern but infections leading cause of death; organism depends on time elapsed since transplantation: first month bacterial processes (wound, urine, lung); 1 to 6 months viral (CMV, EBV) and opportunistic (PCP, Aspergillus); beyond 6 months resemble general community
  - Classic signs of infection such as fever often masked by immunosuppression
  - Pancreatitis and hepatotoxicity due to viral infection or medications
  - Posttransplant malignancies: lymphoproliferative disorder (PTLD), Kaposi sarcoma
  - Steroid-induced diabetes, avascular necrosis, osteoporosis
  - Hyperlipidemia and accelerated atherosclerosis
  - Adrenal axis suppression
  - Medication interactions and potential toxicity: metabolism of immunosuppressive agents often affected by antibiotics, antifungal agents, antituberculosis drugs, anticonvulsants, antacids, histamine blockers, calcium channel blockers

- **Essentials of Management**
  - Continue prophylactic antibiotics and antiviral medications
  - Aggressively treat suspected or identified infections
  - If life-threatening infection present, discontinue immunosuppressive regimen despite risk of graft rejection
  - "Stress" dose steroids required in acutely ill patient recently on corticosteroids as part of immunosuppression regimen
  - Evaluate for drug–drug interactions and monitor for toxicity when adding new medications
  - Biopsy of transplanted organ required for diagnosis of rejection; may require additional immunosuppressive agents
  - If PTLD suspected, reduction of immunosuppression indicated combined with acyclovir or ganciclovir

- **Pearl**

Graft-versus-host disease, although most commonly associated with bone marrow transplantation, can also be seen in intestinal and multivisceral transplantations.

Reference

Dunn DL: Hazardous crossing: immunosuppression and nosocomial infections in solid organ transplant recipients. Surg Infect 2001;2:103. [PMID: 12594865]

3

Ethical Issues

Brain Death

■ Essentials of Diagnosis
- Irreversible cessation of brain function, cortical and brain stem
- Brain stem: no oculocephalic reflex, pupils fixed, lack of motor reflexes, absence of spontaneous respiration
- No spontaneous breathing for 10 minutes after discontinuing mechanical ventilation (patient given 100% O_2 to breathe) and/or $Paco_2 > 55$ mm Hg
- Local or institutional policy may require determination by neurologist or neurosurgeon, need more than one examiner, require two examinations conducted at a defined interval, or mandate electroencephalogram (EEG)

■ Differential Diagnosis
- Hypothermia
- Presence of sedative-hypnotic drugs (benzodiazepines, barbiturates, etc.).
- Severe vegetative state (some brain stem function)

■ Treatment
- Determine if brain death is present by institutional or local criteria
- According to institutional procedure, determine and act accordingly if patient is potential organ donor
- If brain death declaration is made, time of death is time determination made
- Remove life support therapy after declaration of death, except for organ donation

■ Pearl
When testing for apnea, give 100% oxygen through the endotracheal tube to avoid hypoxic injury, then observe for at least 10 minutes or until the $Paco_2$ rises above 60 mm Hg.

Reference

Wijdicks EF: The diagnosis of brain death. N Engl J Med 2001;344:1215. [PMID: 11309637]

Do-Not-Resuscitate Orders (DNR)

- **Essential Concepts**
  - The Do-Not-Resuscitate (Do-Not-Attempt Resuscitation; DNR) order stops automatic cardiopulmonary resuscitation
  - Only applies to patient at time of cardiopulmonary arrest; withholding or withdrawing other care separate decisions
  - DNR extends patient's autonomy to make informed choice, while knowing consequences of decision
  - In multiple organ failure or critical illness, cardiopulmonary resuscitation < 10% likelihood of success and very poor outcome (<5% normal function)
  - Resuscitation of acute, reversible, witnessed arrest often more successful

- **Essentials of Management**
  - Consider DNR discussion with patient or other decision maker for all critically ill patients in ICU
  - Determine if DNR already addressed in advance directives
  - Assure patient and family that DNR does not discontinue comfort measures and pain control
  - Follow institution's DNR policy for documentation; include time of discussion, persons who participated, level of understanding of patient, other decisions about patient care
  - If disagreement about DNR, make efforts to clarify misunderstandings, misconceptions, concerns
  - DNR may be temporarily suspended for general anesthesia or cardiac catheterization, during which there is increased risk of cardiopulmonary arrest

- **Pearl**

Only about 30% of patients with likely very poor outcome have DNR orders.

Reference

Burns JP et al: Do-not-resuscitate order after 25 years. Crit Care Med 2003;31:1543. [PMID: 12771631]

Medical Ethics

- ■ Essential Concepts
  - • Ethical decisions based on four basic principles
  - • Autonomy: Patient has right to make informed decisions and re-
    fusals, if has capacity to understand consequences of decisions;
    capacity means understanding consequences of decision
  - • Beneficence: Care must achieve good not harm; goals of med-
    icine are saving life, prolonging life, relieving suffering, curing
    disease
  - • Nonmaleficence: Avoid harm while meeting other goals and
    principles; at times, may conflict with beneficence
  - • Justice: Treat fairly in relationship to others; allocate resources
    where likely to do most good

- ■ Essentials of Management
  - • Let patients or other decision makers make autonomous deci-
    sions but only after giving sufficient information and confirm-
    ing understanding
  - • Care must focus on achieving goals of medicine
  - • All options and decisions must weigh benefits against risks for
    each diagnostic or therapeutic intervention
  - • Physicians responsible to individual patient; may conflict at
    times with responsibility to community (eg, costs of care, lim-
    ited resources)
  - • Common conflicts: Patient has autonomy to make informed
    choices, but physicians must not allow them to harm themselves.
    When striving to relieve suffering (pain), analgesia may shorten
    life. Patients have right to make decisions, even if they conflict
    with family members

- ■ Pearl

*Designated surrogate decision makers often do not make same deci-
sion as the patient would; prior discussion and communication greatly
improve agreement.*

Reference

Henig NR et al: Biomedical ethics and the withdrawal of advanced life support. Annu Rev Med 2001;52:79. [PMID: 11160769]

Medicolegal Principles

- **Essential Concepts**
    - A patient with capacity to understand consequences may choose or refuse medical care offered
    - Capacity to make medical decisions may be present even without capacity to make other decisions (e.g., financial)
    - Informed consent: Patient consents after understanding benefits, risks, and their likelihood for a test or treatment
    - Informed denial (refusal): Patient declines a test or procedure, but only after demonstrating understanding the consequences of refusal
    - When patient lacks capacity, use surrogate decision maker, often, but not always, a family member; ideally chosen in advance by patient
    - Surrogate must decide based on patient's likely choice, either explicit or implicit
    - In absence of surrogate, may need to make a "best interests" decision—what would a reasonable person choose?

- **Essentials of Management**
    - Evaluate capacity as patient's ability to understand consequences of individual medical choices presented
    - For informed consent, explain likely events, consequences, results; very rare events need not be mentioned
    - Always make a judgment about the patient's level of understanding, whether consenting to or declining offered treatment
    - If a surrogate does not know patient's wishes, make a "best interest" decision weighing benefits and burdens of treatment to patient
    - In absence of any surrogate who knows patient's wishes, physicians may make decisions according to local policy, including forgoing of treatment.

- **Pearl**

Forgoing treatment in the absence of clear-cut direct knowledge that this is the patient's wish can still be undertaken.

Reference

Meisel A et al: Seven legal barriers to end-of-life care: myths, realities, and grains of truth. JAMA 2000;284:2495. [PMID: 11074780]

Withholding & Withdrawing Care

- Essential Concepts
  - Any medical care may be withdrawn or withheld, not just extraordinary measures
  - Under no obligation to provide care that does not meet a goal of medicine—prolonging life, relieving suffering, or curing disease
  - Patient with capacity to make decisions can ask that care be withdrawn or withheld
  - Advance directive may designate withholding of treatment
  - Not helpful to distinguish ordinary (feeding, hydration, pain medication) from extraordinary care (mechanical ventilation, major surgery, blood transfusions)
  - Extensive discussions with patient, family, and staff essential for decisions regarding forgoing care
  - Always maintain patient comfort, dignity, hygiene

- Essentials of Management
  - Patient or surrogate decision maker asks that care be withheld or withdrawn
  - Physician believes current or proposed care not indicated because of very low likelihood of benefit
  - Risks of current or proposed care outweigh potential benefit; such care conflicts with prolonging life or relieving suffering
  - If forgoing of treatment decided, follow institutional policy for documenting in medical record; include date and time of discussion, persons who participated (patient, family members, surrogate decision makers), level of understanding of patient
  - Involve ICU staff in decision-making process; inform of decisions
  - Continue comfort measures, including adequate analgesia and sedation
  - Reassess patient's wishes periodically

- Pearl

A patient or surrogate may be unaware of the option to withhold or withdraw care.

Reference

Nyman DJ Sprung CL: End-of-life decision making in the intensive care unit. Intensive Care Med 2000;26:1414. [PMID: 11126250]

4

Bleeding & Transfusions

Bleeding in the Critically Ill Patient

- **Essentials of Diagnosis**
  - Spontaneous bleeding or bleeding from invasive procedures due to one or more defects in hemostasis
  - Normal hemostasis needs intact vascular endothelium, coagulation factors, adequate platelet number and function
  - Thrombocytopenia or platelet dysfunction: ecchymoses and mucosal bleeding, posttraumatic or surgical bleeding
  - Acquired or inherited coagulopathies: spontaneous hemarthroses or soft tissue hematomas
  - Severe coagulopathy, thrombocytopenia, or disseminated intravascular coagulation (DIC): generalized bleeding, especially new acute onset
  - Excessive warfarin: soft tissue hematoma

- **Differential Diagnosis**
  - Abnormal prothrombin time (PT) only: vitamin K deficiency, liver disease, warfarin, specific inhibitor
  - Abnormal activated partial thromboplastin time (aPTT) only: inherited coagulopathy, heparin, lupus anticoagulant, specific inhibitor
  - Both aPTT and PT abnormal: vitamin K deficiency, DIC, liver disease, heparin or warfarin
  - Abnormal aPTT, PTT, platelet count: DIC (microangiopathic hemolytic anemia, low fibrinogen, elevated fibrin degradation products, elevated D-dimer)
  - Screening tests normal: platelet dysfunction, endothelial damage, factor XIII deficiency

- **Treatment**
  - Assess severity and acuity of bleeding; estimate rapidity of blood loss; treat if active or anticipated bleeding, invasive procedures necessary
  - Management depends on etiology; vitamin K, fresh frozen plasma, cryoprecipitate, platelet transfusions, stopping anticoagulants

- **Pearl**

Consider acute acquired dysfunction of platelets if unexplained bleeding with no previous history; may be due to renal failure, drugs such as aspirin, NSAIDs, or platelet inhibitors.

Reference

DeSancho MT et al: Bleeding and thrombotic complications in critically ill patients with cancer. Crit Care Clin 2001;17:599. [PMID: 11525050]

Coagulopathy, Acquired

- **Essentials of Diagnosis**
  - Excessive or prolonged bleeding from punctures, incisions, GI tract, mucosal membranes, joints, retroperitoneal space, other sites
  - Abnormal coagulation time (prothrombin time [PT] or activated partial thromboplastin time [aPTT]) in absence of inherited coagulopathy
  - Causes: warfarin, heparin administration; liver disease; vitamin K deficiency (malnutrition, antibiotics, poor intake); disseminated intravascular coagulation (sepsis, hypotension, release of bone marrow thromboplastins, liver injury, abruptio placenta, amniotic fluid embolism), trauma (fat embolism, brain injury); acquired circulating anticoagulant (antibody to coagulation factor)

- **Differential Diagnosis**
  - Inherited coagulopathy
  - Thrombocytopenia or qualitative platelet disorder, vitamin C deficiency
  - Abnormal aPTT without increased risk of bleeding (lupus anticoagulant)

- **Treatment**
  - Establish etiology
  - Treat if active bleeding, high risk for bleeding, anticipated procedure (lumbar puncture, central venous catheter, surgery)
  - Vitamin K, 1–10 mg orally or subcutaneously, if vitamin K deficiency suspected
  - Replace factors if moderate to severe bleeding; fresh frozen plasma (FFP) contains factors absent in liver disease, vitamin K deficiency, warfarin treatment, DIC; give FFP equal to 50% of plasma volume (20 mL/kg ideal body weight); one unit FFP approximately 250–300 mL, so give 4–6 units FFP over 6–12 hours

- **Pearl**

Many antibiotics destroy enteric bacteria, which produce vitamin K; give weekly vitamin K to ICU patients who are receiving antibiotics.

Reference

Teitel JM: Clinical approach to the patient with unexpected bleeding. Clin Lab Haematol 2000;22 (1 Suppl):9. [PMID: 11251652]

Coagulopathy, Inherited

- **Essentials of Diagnosis**
  - Excessive or prolonged bleeding from punctures, incisions, GI tract, mucosal membranes, joints, retroperitoneal space, other sites
  - History of lifelong abnormal bleeding or family history of bleeding disorders
  - Abnormally prolonged coagulation time (prothrombin time [PT] or activated partial thromboplastin time [aPTT])
  - Common: von Willebrand disease (autosomal dominant deficiency of von Willebrand factor with qualitative platelet dysfunction and prolonged aPTT due to factor VIII deficiency); hemophilia A (sex-linked, variably dysfunctional factor VIII); hemophilia B (sex-linked deficiency of active factor IX).
  - Rare: deficiency of factors II, V, VII, X, XI, XIII, fibrinogen
  - Inheritance of gene coding abnormal coagulation factor or insufficient production of a factor; X-linked or autosomal

- **Differential Diagnosis**
  - Acquired coagulopathy
  - Thrombocytopenia or qualitative platelet disorder, vitamin C deficiency
  - Abnormal aPTT without risk of bleeding (lupus anticoagulant)

- **Treatment**
  - Establish etiology
  - Treat if active bleeding, high risk for bleeding, anticipated invasive procedure (lumbar puncture, central venous catheter, surgery)
  - von Willebrand disease: desmopressin (intravenous or intranasal), cryoprecipitate
  - VIII deficiency: desmopressin for mild bleeding, purified or recombinant factor VIII
  - IX deficiency: Purified or recombinant factor IX
  - Fresh frozen plasma contains factors VIII, IX, most other factors, but should not be used unless others not available

- **Pearl**

A woman with a hereditary coagulopathy almost always has von Willebrand disease.

Reference

Bolton-Maggs PH et al: Haemophilias A and B. Lancet 2003;361:1801. [PMID: 12781551]

Heparin-Induced Thrombocytopenia (HIT)

- ■ Essentials of Diagnosis
    - • Unexplained arterial or venous thrombosis, pulmonary embolism, stroke, coronary occlusion, upper extremity DVT, with fall in platelet count 4–14 days after starting heparin
    - • Occurs with both therapeutic and prophylactic heparin, including heparin flushing of catheters; may occur after heparin stopped
    - • Type I: slight fall in platelet count in 10–20% with unfractionated heparin; nonimmune mediated, no clinical consequence, earlier onset
    - • Type II: 1% given unfractionated heparin, 0.3% low molecular weight heparin, severe immune-mediated, associated with thrombosis (often arterial), later onset (unless due to re-exposure to heparin)
    - • In type II, heparin-platelet factor 4 complex triggers antibody; antibody-antigen complex binds to platelet surface causing aggregation and platelet-rich clots; no risk of bleeding from thrombocytopenia (platelet count usually > 20,000)
    - • Suspect in all patients with thrombocytopenia receiving heparin; especially if rapid return of platelets after heparin stopped

- ■ Differential Diagnosis
    - • Other causes of thrombocytopenia
    - • Warfarin skin necrosis
    - • Other thrombotic states, including malignancies, protein C or S deficiency

- ■ Treatment
    - • Stop all heparin: therapeutic, prophylactic, flushes
    - • Use direct thrombin inhibitor (lepirudin or argatroban) for patients who continue to need anticoagulation, then warfarin; avoid starting warfarin until platelet count > 100,000/μL (may contribute to hypercoagulable state)
    - • Avoid future exposure to heparin

- ■ Pearl

Even small amounts of heparin can cause HIT, even heparin being given to keep intravenous catheters from clotting.

Reference

Walenga JM et al: Heparin-induced thrombocytopenia, paradoxical thromboembolism, and other adverse effects of heparin-type therapy. Hematol Oncol Clin North Am 2003;17:259. [PMID: 12627671]

Plasma Transfusions

■ Essential Concepts

- Fresh frozen plasma (FFP) replaces coagulation factors in acquired or inherited coagulopathy (liver disease, vitamin K deficiency, DIC, warfarin therapy, hemophilia A or B, other inherited coagulopathies; antithrombin deficiency); also for plasma exchange therapy
- Cryoprecipitate replaces fibrinogen, factor VIII; cryoprecipitate-poor plasma useful for TTP/HUS
- Plasma transfusion not indicated for volume expansion or treatment of hypovolemic shock, hypoalbuminemia

■ Essentials of Management

- Treat underlying disorder
- Assess need for FFP: active bleeding, anticipated bleeding from invasive procedure, severe coagulopathy, effect of alternative therapy (vitamin K), response to discontinuing warfarin
- FFP requirement for coagulopathy based on increasing coagulation factors > 50% of normal; assume patient has 0% factors to start
- Give volume of FFP equal to 50% of plasma volume (20 mL/kg ideal body weight); each FFP unit approximately 250–300 mL; therefore, provide 4–6 units FFP over 6–12 hours, depending on patient tolerance to volume replacement and urgency of bleeding
- Coagulation factors effective in circulation 4–24 hours, depending on factor
- For TTP/HUS, use cryoprecipitate-free FFP for TTP/HUS during plasmapheresis; to replace fibrinogen in DIC and hypofibrinogenemia, use cryoprecipitate
- Complications of plasma therapy: volume overload, infection

■ Pearl

In patients with severe liver disease, FFP transfusions will almost never completely "correct" the coagulopathy; avoid fluid overload by limiting total transfused.

Reference

Hellstern P et al: Practical guidelines for the clinical use of plasma. Thromb Res 2002;107 (1 Suppl):S53. [PMID: 12379294]

Qualitative Platelet Dysfunction

- **Essentials of Diagnosis**
  - Mucosal bleeding, ecchymoses, or surgical bleeding
  - Platelet count $> 50,000$ per mm^3
  - May have abnormal bleeding time
  - Inherited or acquired condition or medication associated with qualitative platelet dysfunction
  - Acquired common; medications (aspirin, NSAIDs, dextran, glycoprotein IIb/IIIa inhibitors, ticlopidine, clopidogrel), uremia, recent cardiopulmonary bypass
  - Inherited rare; lifelong history of bleeding, normal platelet count; defects may be in adhesion (Bernard-Soulier syndrome), aggregation (Glanzmann disease or glycoprotein IIB/IIIa deficiency), release of platelet components, or decreased platelet factor 3

- **Differential Diagnosis**
  - Thrombocytopenia
  - Coagulopathies (normal bleeding time)
  - Disseminated intravascular coagulation with thrombocytopenia
  - Severe vitamin C deficiency

- **Treatment**
  - Determine risk of or severity of bleeding
  - Discontinue potentially responsible medications
  - Avoid invasive procedures
  - If bleeding, intravenous desmopressin acetate may improve platelet function
  - Renal failure patients may benefit from hemodialysis
  - Platelet transfusions may be tried in cases of persistent severe bleeding due to drugs, inherited platelet dysfunction

- **Pearl**

Measuring bleeding time may not be helpful because of poor correlation between bleeding time and risk of bleeding from platelet disorders.

Reference

George JN: Platelets. Lancet 2000;355:1531. [PMID: 10801186]

Thrombocytopenia

- ■ Essentials of Diagnosis
  - • Platelet count < 50,000; petechiae or ecchymoses, or mild to severe mucosal membrane or intracranial bleeding
  - • Decreased production (bone marrow infiltration by infection or malignancy, toxins, alcohol, drugs, aplastic anemia); increased destruction (idiopathic, DIC, drugs, hypersplenism, heparin-associated thrombocytopenia, HELLP syndrome)
  - • Spontaneous bleeding when platelet count < 20,000, but highly variable; for same platelet count, platelet destruction less bleeding than low production; qualitative platelet dysfunction worsens bleeding

- ■ Differential Diagnosis
  - • Pseudothrombocytopenia (platelet clumping *in vitro* due to EDTA anticoagulant)
  - • Nonthrombocytopenic disorders of hemostasis (coagulopathy, vascular injury)
  - • Vasculitis with palpable nonthrombocytopenic purpura
  - • Thrombotic thrombocytopenic purpura (TTP) not associated with increased bleeding

- ■ Treatment
  - • Transfuse if < 50,000/μL and major surgical procedure planned; < 30,000/μL, minor surgery or spontaneous bleeding; < 5000–10,000, prophylactically
  - • Transfuse at higher count if bleeding, fever, infection, renal failure, platelet dysfunction, low production (bone marrow failure); at lower counts if platelet destruction (transfusions minimally useful); transfusion contraindicated in TTP/HUS, heparin-induced thrombocytopenia
  - • Type-specific random-donor platelets, 6–8 units; expect 5000–10,000/μL increase per unit
  - • Complications: volume overload, infections, sensitization to platelets with decreased transfusion effectiveness
  - • Other therapy: idiopathic thrombocytopenic purpura (corticosteroids, IgG); renal failure, von Willebrand disease (desmopressin), anemia (red cell transfusions)

- ■ Pearl
  If platelet count does not rise by 5000–10,000 for each unit of platelets, suspect platelet destruction, such as ITP.

Reference

Drews RE, Weinberger SE: Thrombocytopenic disorders in critically ill patients. Am J Respir Crit Care Med 2000; 162:347. PMID: 10934051

Transfusion of Red Blood Cells

- **Essential Concepts**
  - Anemia adversely affects oxygen delivery to organs, increases risk of bleeding; may be acute (blood loss, hemolysis, decreased production) or chronic (underlying disease)
  - Transfusion of red blood cells (RBC) indicated for anemia plus limited oxygen delivery, organ ischemia (myocardial infarction, unstable angina), likelihood of future blood loss, symptomatic anemia
  - For patients with acute recurrent bleeding, anticipate need for RBC transfusions and maintain Hgb approximately 10 g/100 mL
  - RBC transfusion not indicated for stable mild anemia (Hgb > 8–10 g/100 mL), if no evidence of impaired O_2 delivery, no myocardial ischemia, recent myocardial infarction, shock, hypotension

- **Essentials of Management**
  - Provide specific treatment for anemia (iron, folate, vitamin B_{12}, epoetin alfa)
  - Transfuse homologous packed RBC; expect Hgb rise 0.5–1 g/100 mL per unit (if no ongoing loss)
  - Leukocyte-poor RBCs limit nonhemolytic transfusion reaction and HLA sensitization for potential transplant recipients; washed RBCs for patients sensitive to plasma components
  - Number of transfused RBC units depends on hemodynamic stability, ongoing losses, changes in intravascular volume, bone marrow response
  - Multiple transfusions associated with thrombocytopenia, coagulation factor deficiency; rarely citrate intoxication, hyperkalemia, hypothermia
  - Complications: transfusion reactions (fever, anaphylaxis, hemolysis, alloimmunization); volume overload (especially with heart failure, renal failure); infections (hepatitis B and C, HIV, CMV)

- **Pearl**

Unnecessary RBC transfusions associated with worse ICU outcome; may be due to increased immunosuppression.

Reference

Hebert PC, et al: A multicenter, randomized, controlled clinical trial of transfusion requirements in critical care. Transfusion Requirements in Critical Care Investigators, Canadian Critical Care Trials Group. N Engl J Med 1999;340:409. [PMID: 9971864]

Transfusion Reactions

- **Essentials of Diagnosis**
  - \> 90% acute reactions nonhemolytic: fever, lung injury (infiltrates, hypoxemia over 1–4 days), allergic (urticaria, fever, rash, pruritis, bronchospasm, anaphylaxis); 1–3% of transfusions
  - Acute hemolysis < 10%; back, joint pain, chills, fever, hypotension, tachycardia; acute renal failure, cardiovascular collapse, DIC; from transfusion of incompatible blood with recipient antibodies to donor cells or donor antibodies to recipient cells
  - Chronic reactions > 1 week; antibodies to non-ABO antigens; may be subclinical (unable to find subsequent compatible donor blood by crossmatching) or mild antibody-mediated hemolysis
  - Nonspecific complications of transfusions: hyperkalemia, circulatory overload, hypothermia, hypocalcemia, thrombocytopenia, immunosuppression, infections

- **Differential Diagnosis**
  - Infection and sepsis
  - Allergic reaction to medications
  - Pulmonary edema
  - Other causes of hemolysis

- **Treatment**
  - Stop transfusion immediately to minimize incompatible blood administered; assess severity, type of reaction
  - Send remainder of blood and patient sample for repeat crossmatching; check for hemolysis (blood smear, bilirubin, haptoglobin, free hemoglobin), DIC
  - Hemolytic reaction: intravascular volume expansion to maintain renal perfusion; diuretics to maintain urine output
  - Minor nonhemolytic reactions in patient requiring multiple repeated transfusions: decide whether repeat evaluation needed; antipyretics prior to transfusions

- **Pearl**

Transfusion-related acute lung injury (TRALI) is caused by donor antibodies; "high-risk" donors can sometimes be identified.

Reference

Goodnough LT, et al: Transfusion medicine. First of two parts—blood transfusion. N Engl J Med 1999;340:438. [PMID: 9971869]

Warfarin Overdose

- **Essentials of Diagnosis**
  - History of coumadin therapy or known overdose
  - Prolonged prothrombin time, expressed as international normalized ratio, INR > 5
  - May or may not have clinical bleeding

- **Differential Diagnosis**
  - Congenital coagulopathy
  - Acquired coagulopathy
  - Heparin

- **Treatment**
  - Treat if serious bleed into critical area (intracranial), active bleeding, severe anemia, high risk for future bleeding, anticipated invasive procedure (lumbar puncture, central venous catheter, surgery)
  - INR > therapeutic and < 5.0; no significant bleeding: Lower or omit dose; resume therapy at lower dose when INR therapeutic
  - INR > 5.0, < 9.0; no significant bleeding: Omit next 1–2 doses, resume at lower dose when INR therapeutic; vitamin K_1 (1–2.5 mg orally); if patient at increased risk for bleeding; give vitamin K_1 (2–4 mg orally)
  - INR > 9.0; no significant bleeding; omit warfarin; vitamin K_1 (3–5 mg orally)
  - INR > 20; serious bleeding. Omit warfarin; vitamin K_1 (10 mg, slow IV infusion) plus fresh plasma; repeat vitamin K_1 every 12 h.
  - Life-threatening bleeding: Omit warfarin; prothrombin complex concentrate and vitamin K_1 (10 mg, slow IV infusion); repeat if necessary, depending on INR
  - Patients who need anticoagulation (prosthetic valve, atrial fibrillation, deep venous thrombosis, etc.) should have anticoagulation restarted when safe

- **Pearl**

Without severe bleeding and INR < 9, low-dose oral vitamin K usually returns INR to therapeutic range quickly and safely.

Reference

Crowther MA et al: Oral vitamin K lowers the international normalized ratio more rapidly than subcutaneous vitamin K in the treatment of warfarin-associated coagulopathy. A randomized, controlled trial. Ann Intern Med 2002;137:251. [PMID: 12186515]

Warfarin Skin Necrosis

- **■ Essentials of Diagnosis**
  - Painful petechiae beginning 2–6 days after starting warfarin; may progress to demarcated ecchymosis, bullae, and skin necrosis
  - Seen most often over subcutaneous fat of buttocks, breasts, abdomen; more common in women
  - Rare (0.01–0.1%), very serious complication of warfarin
  - Suspect in patients with rapid increase in INR with early doses of warfarin, hypercoagulable states (deficiency of proteins C or S, heparin-induced thrombocytopenia, resistance to activated protein C), previous complications suspected to be warfarin skin necrosis
  - Starting warfarin may lead to transient decrease in anticoagulant proteins C and S (short half-lives) while procoagulant factors (factor Xa) not reduced; imbalance favors coagulation and thrombosis; imbalance more likely with deficiency of naturally occurring anticoagulants

- **■ Differential Diagnosis**
  - Disseminated intravascular coagulation with purpura fulminans
  - Necrotizing fasciitis
  - Arterial or venous insufficiency
  - Vasculitis

- **■ Treatment**
  - Stop warfarin
  - Administer vitamin K, fresh frozen plasma
  - Use alternative method of anticoagulation, such as heparin, if necessary
  - May need skin debridement
  - Prevention: use low starting dosages of warfarin, usually 5 mg orally daily; overlap with heparin therapy

- **■ Pearl**

If INR rapidly rises after the first dose of warfarin, watch patient closely for signs of skin necrosis.

Reference

Ansell J et al: Managing oral anticoagulant therapy. Chest 2001;119(1 Suppl):22S. [PMID: 11157641]

5

Fluids, Electrolytes, & Acid-Base

Hypercalcemia

■ **Essentials of Diagnosis**

- Serum calcium $[Ca^{2+}] > 10.5$ mg/dL (corrected for albumin) or elevated ionized calcium
- Anorexia, nausea, vomiting, adynamic ileus, constipation, abdominal pain, pancreatitis
- Altered mental status with apathy, obtundation, coma, psychosis
- Polyuria, polydipsia, nephrocalcinosis, impaired urinary concentrating ability
- Band keratopathy of eyes
- Increased risk of bone fractures
- ECG with shortened QT interval; cardiac arrhythmias especially in patients on digitalis

■ **Differential Diagnosis**

- Hyperparathyroidism
- Vitamin A or D intoxication
- Milk-alkali syndrome
- Adrenal insufficiency
- Paget disease of bone
- Familial hypocalciuric hypercalcemia
- Granulomatous diseases: sarcoidosis, tuberculosis, fungal infections
- Malignancy
- Thiazide diuretics
- Thyrotoxicosis
- Immobilization

■ **Treatment**

- Aggressive fluid resuscitation with normal saline
- Once euvolemic, loop diuretics to induce calciuresis; avoid thiazides
- Calcitonin useful with life-threatening hypercalcemia in initial phase of therapy due to rapid onset of action but transient effect
- Bisphosphonates lower calcium over several days
- Glucocorticoids effective in steroid-sensitive malignancy, granulomatous disease, vitamin D induced hypercalcemia
- Hemodialysis
- Evaluate for underlying etiology especially malignancy

■ **Pearl**

The serum calcium level should be corrected according to the patient's albumin level based on the following calculation:
$$calcium_{measured} + 0.8 \times (4 - albumin).$$

Reference

Fukugawa M et al: Calcium homeostasis and imbalance. Nephron 2002;92:41.
[PMID: 12425329]

Hypocalcemia

- **Essentials of Diagnosis**
  - Serum calcium $[Ca^{2+}] < 8.5$ mg/dL (corrected for albumin) or reduced ionized calcium
  - Correction for albumin: $calcium_{measured} + 0.8 \times (4 - albumin)$
  - Symptoms correlate with rapidity and magnitude of fall
  - Tetany, paresthesias, hyperreflexia most common manifestations; acute hyperventilation may evoke tetany
  - Altered mental status, seizures, muscle weakness, papilledema
  - Chvostek sign: tapping facial nerve leads to grimace
  - Trousseau sign: inflating blood pressure cuff causes carpopedal spasm of outstretched hand
  - Reduced myocardial contractility can precipitate congestive heart failure
  - ECG with prolonged QT interval; ventricular arrhythmias

- **Differential Diagnosis**
  - Chronic renal failure
  - Hypomagnesemia
  - Acute pancreatitis
  - Following parathyroidectomy
  - Acute hyperphosphatemia
  - Septic shock
  - Hypoparathyroidism, pseudohypoparathyroidism
  - Vitamin D deficiency or malabsorption
  - Rhabdomyolysis, tumor lysis syndrome
  - Medications: loop diuretics, aminoglycosides
  - Massive blood transfusion due to citrate

- **Treatment**
  - Intravenous calcium for acute symptoms; avoid if serum phosphate elevated due to risk of calcium-phosphate precipitation
  - Oral calcium between meals with vitamin D supplementation
  - Thiazide diuretics may be considered to prevent hypercalciuria
  - Correct hypomagnesemia
  - Address underlying etiology
  - Anticonvulsants may be used to treat seizures but may exacerbate hypocalcemia by increasing vitamin D metabolism

- **Pearl**

When hypocalcemia develops immediately after a subtotal parathyroidectomy, it may be due to a stunned parathyroid gland with transient hypoparathyroidism or hungry-bone syndrome. In hungry-bone syndrome, serum phosphate is decreased while it is elevated in hypoparathyroidism.

Reference

Carlstedt F et al: Hypocalcemic syndromes. Crit Care Clin 2001;17:139. [PMID: 11219226]

Hyperkalemia

- **Essentials of Diagnosis**
  - Serum potassium [K^+] level > 5 mEq/L
  - Weakness beginning in legs, paresthesias, hyporeflexia
  - ECG changes occur at plasma [K^+] > 5.7 mEq/L with peaked T-waves; subsequent ECG progression: reduced P-wave amplitude, PR prolongation, QRS widening, broad sine waves, ventricular fibrillation
  - Transtubular potassium gradient (TTKG) can differentiate renal from nonrenal causes: Urine/Plasma (K^+) × Plasma/Urine (Osm); product < 6 renal or hypoaldosterone effect; > 10 nonrenal

- **Differential Diagnosis**
  - Excess intake: potassium supplements or salts
  - Reduced excretion: renal failure, adrenal insufficiency, hypoaldosteronism, type IV renal tubular acidosis
  - Intracellular shift: acidosis, rhabdomyolysis, tumor lysis, severe hemolysis, burns
  - Factitious: hemolysis of blood sample, extreme leukocytosis or thrombocytosis
  - Medications: K^+-sparing diuretics, ACE-inhibitors, beta-blockers, succinylcholine, penicillin VK, trimethoprim-sulfamethoxazole

- **Treatment**
  - Calcium gluconate or chloride solution: immediate cardioprotective effect; drug of choice with acute ECG changes
  - Bicarbonate shifts potassium intracellularly, especially if acidemic
  - Nebulized beta-agonist albuterol can decrease [K^+] by 0.6 mEq/L within 1 hour
  - Insulin shifts potassium intracellularly and should be given along with dextrose infusion
  - Binding resin kayexalate removes potassium enterally; use cautiously in constipation as may develop concretions
  - Loop diuretics lower body potassium over hours
  - Hemodialysis most reliable and efficient method in reducing total body potassium
  - Limit potassium in diet, intravenous fluids, medications

- **Pearl**

Attempts made to correct hyperkalemia in the setting of acidosis may result in significant total body potassium depletion and serum hypokalemia once acidosis is resolved.

Reference

Kim HJ et al: Therapeutic approach to hyperkalemia. Nephron 2002;92:33. [PMID: 12401936]

Hypokalemia

- **Essentials of Diagnosis**
  - Serum potassium $[K^+] < 3.5$ mEq/L
  - Usually asymptomatic
  - Muscle weakness, respiratory failure, paralysis, paresthesias, ileus, postural hypotension
  - Exacerbates hepatic encephalopathy
  - Transtubular potassium gradient (TTKG) can differentiate renal from nonrenal causes: Urine/Plasma $[K^+] \times$ Plasma/Urine (Osm); product > 4 renal loss or hyperaldosterone effect; < 2 gastrointestinal loss
  - ECG with flattened T-waves, ST depression, U-waves; arrhythmias include premature ventricular beats, ventricular tachycardia, ventricular fibrillation

- **Differential Diagnosis**
  - Renal losses: hyperaldosteronism, glucocorticoid excess, licorice ingestion, osmotic diuresis, renal tubular acidosis (I, II), hypomagnesemia; Fanconi, Bartter, Gitelman, Liddle syndromes
  - Extrarenal losses: severe diarrhea, nasogastric suctioning, sweating
  - Intracellular shift: alkalosis, insulin, hypokalemic periodic paralysis
  - Medications: loop diuretics, thiazides, carbenicillin, amphotericin B, cisplatin, aminoglycosides
  - Inadequate intake

- **Treatment**
  - Oral and intravenous replacement; oral supplementation preferred because parenteral replacement rate limited by local irritation; central venous catheter infusions may lead to high intracardiac levels precipitating arrhythmias
  - Cautiously replace in patients with renal impairment
  - Magnesium replacement essential as hypokalemia may be refractory until magnesium level in normal range
  - Goal potassium level > 4 mEq/L in acute myocardial infarction when prone to hypokalemia-related arrhythmias
  - Correct underlying etiologies whenever possible

- **Pearl**

As a rule of thumb, replacing 10 mEq/L of potassium (oral or intravenous) will increase serum potassium levels by 0.1 mEq/L.

Reference

Kim GH et al: Therapeutic approach to hypokalemia. Nephron 2002;92:28. [PMID: 12401935]

Hypermagnesemia

■ Essentials of Diagnosis
- Serum magnesium $[Mg^{++}] > 2.7$ mg/dL
- Reduced deep-tendon reflexes
- May progress to respiratory muscle failure
- Hypotension with reduced vascular resistance
- Somnolence and coma with extremely elevated levels
- Decreased serum calcium may be seen
- Progression of ECG changes: interventricular conduction delay, prolonged QT interval, heart block, asystole
- Generally occurs with renal insufficiency and excessive intake
- Other risk factors: nephrotoxic agents, hypotension or hypovolemia with oliguria, preeclampsia-eclampsia receiving large therapeutic doses

■ Differential Diagnosis
- Renal failure: acute and chronic
- Excess ingestion: antacids, laxatives
- Intravenous administration: parenteral nutrition, intravenous fluids

■ Treatment
- Eliminate infusion of all magnesium-containing compounds
- Intravenous calcium gluconate or chloride reverses acute cardiovascular toxicity and respiratory failure
- Hemodialysis with magnesium-free dialysate
- Monitor deep tendon reflexes when treating with "therapeutic hypermagnesemia" as in obstetric patients
- Correct renal insufficiency

■ Pearl

Magnesium can be thought of as "nature's calcium channel blocker."

Reference

Topf JM: Hypomagnesemia and hypermagnesemia. Rev Endocr Metab Disord 2003;4:195. [PMID: 12766548]

Hypomagnesemia

- **Essentials of Diagnosis**
  - Serum magnesium $[Mg^{++}] < 1.7$ mg/dL
  - Weakness, muscle cramps, tremor, tetany, altered mental status
  - Positive Babinski response
  - May occur with acute myocardial infarction; increases risk of arrhythmias including atrial and ventricular tachycardias; *torsade de pointes*
  - Associated with hypokalemia, hypocalcemia, metabolic alkalosis

- **Differential Diagnosis**
  - Excessive diuresis: postobstructive, osmotic, resolving ATN
  - Malabsorption, severe diarrhea
  - Hyperparathyroidism
  - Thyrotoxicosis
  - Alcoholism
  - Drugs: diuretics, amphotericin B, aminoglycosides, cisplatin, cyclosporine, loop diuretics
  - Acute pancreatitis
  - Inadequate nutritional intake
  - Gitelman syndrome

- **Treatment**
  - Serum magnesium level may not reflect total body depletion because most magnesium is intracellular
  - Intravenous magnesium replacement: limit to 50 mmol in 24 hours except in severe life-threatening hypomagnesemia
  - Reduce replacement dose in renal impairment
  - Follow serum levels and deep-tendon reflexes during replacement
  - Address underlying etiology

- **Pearl**

In hypomagnesemia associated hypokalemia and hypocalcemia, magnesium replacement is essential to the correction of the other two electrolytes abnormalities.

Reference

Topf JM: Hypomagnesemia and hypermagnesemia. Rev Endocr Metab Disord 2003;4:195. [PMID: 12766548]

Hypernatremia

- **Essentials of Diagnosis**
  - Serum sodium $[Na^+] > 145$ mEq/L associated with hypertonicity
  - Altered mentation, impaired cognition, loss of consciousness
  - Thirst present if mentation preserved
  - Polyuria suggests diabetes insipidus
  - Elderly living in chronic care facilities with dementia and decreased access to water constitute highly susceptible group
  - Free water deficit: depletion of total body water (TBW) relative to total body solute
  - Evaluate urine osmolality, serum osmolality, responsiveness to antidiuretic hormone administration

- **Differential Diagnosis**
  - Inadequate water intake: decreased access to water, impaired thirst response
  - Excessive nonrenal hypotonic water loss: vomiting, diarrhea, sweating
  - Water diuresis: diabetes insipidus (central or nephrogenic)
  - Exogenous solute administration: hypertonic saline, sodium bicarbonate, glucose, mannitol, feeding solutions

- **Treatment**
  - Estimate free water deficit: $TBW_{patient} \times [([Na^+]_{patient} - [Na^+]_{normal})/[Na^+]_{normal}]$
  - Rate of correction depends on acuity of onset of hypernatremia; in general, recommended to be 10 mEq/L per day
  - Excessively rapid replacement of free water may lead to cerebral edema
  - Volume resuscitation with normal saline
  - Once euvolemic, correction of hypernatremia changed to hypotonic fluid replacement
  - Addressing underlying etiology necessary as some causes require specific intervention; central diabetes insipidus treated with desmopressin acetate

- **Pearl**

The presence of polyuria with dilute urine in the face of hypernatremia suggests that excessive water loss is due to the inability to concentrate urine appropriately and is consistent with central or nephrogenic diabetes insipidus.

Reference

Kang SK et al: Pathogenesis and treatment of hypernatremia. Nephron 2002;92:14. [PMID: 12401933]

Hyponatremia

■ Essentials of Diagnosis

- Serum sodium $[Na^+] < 135$ mEq/L
- Generally asymptomatic until serum sodium < 125 mEq/L
- Symptoms related to acuity of change: irritability, nausea, vomiting, headache, lethargy, seizures, coma
- Can be associated with hypertonic, isotonic, and hypotonic states; hypotonic hyponatremia can be seen in clinical situations in which extracellular volume is low, normal, or high
- Comparing serum and urine osmolality and assessing volume status important in identifying etiology

■ Differential Diagnosis

- Hypotonic hypovolemic: vomiting, diarrhea, third-spacing, diuretics (especially thiazides)
- Hypotonic normovolemic: SIADH (associated with pulmonary or CNS disorders), hypothyroidism, adrenal insufficiency, psychogenic polydipsia
- Hypotonic hypervolemic: congestive heart failure, cirrhosis, nephrotic syndrome, protein-losing enteropathy, pregnancy
- Isotonic states: pseudohyponatremia (hyperproteinemia, hyperlipidemia)
- Hypertonic states: hyperglycemia ($[Na^+]$ falls 1.6 mEq/L for each 100 mg/dL increase in glucose), mannitol administration

■ Treatment

- Aggressiveness of correction depends on severity of hyponatremia, acuity of onset, presence of neurological symptoms
- In general, correction should not exceed 8 mEq/L per day
- When hypovolemia present, restoring effective extracellular volume takes priority
- Fluid restriction key in all other forms of hypotonic hyponatremia
- Consider demeclocycline in SIADH
- Combination therapy with hypertonic saline and furosemide reserved for significant neurologic symptoms
- Underlying cause should be addressed and treated

■ Pearl

Excessively rapid correction of sodium (> 20 mEq/L in the first 24 hours) or overcorrection (> 140 mEq/L) may lead to central pontine myelinolysis. Those at highest risk include alcoholics and premenopausal women with acute hyponatremia.

Reference

Halperin ML et al: Clinical approach to disorders of salt and water balance. Crit Care Clin 2002;18:249. [PMID: 12053833]

Hyperphosphatemia

- ■ Essentials of Diagnosis
  - • Serum phosphate > 5 mg/dL
  - • Usually without significant symptoms
  - • Associated hypocalcemia may lead to tetany, seizures, cardiac arrhythmias, hypotension
  - • Complications primarily result from calcium phosphate salt precipitation within solid organs including heart, lung, kidney; heart block from conduction system involvement
  - • Highest risk with acute tissue injury in setting of renal failure

- ■ Differential Diagnosis
  - • Chronic renal failure
  - • Acute renal failure
  - • Hypoparathyroidism
  - • Cellular destruction: rhabdomyolysis, tumor lysis, hemolysis
  - • Excess nutritional intake
  - • Phosphate enemas or bowel preparations

- ■ Treatment
  - • Treatment dependent on symptoms and clinical findings; not on absolute level
  - • Urgent intervention should be considered in presence of heart block or symptomatic hypocalcemia
  - • Discontinue all exogenous sources of phosphate
  - • Normal saline infusion enhances phosphate excretion
  - • Hemodialysis readily removes extracellular phosphate; effect transient due to large intracellular stores
  - • Phosphate-binders given with food are effective chronically
  - • Address underlying etiology

- ■ Pearl

A calcium-phosphate product greater than 70 is predictive of metastatic calcification in various organs and calcium containing phosphate binders should be avoided.

Reference

Malluche HH et al: Hyperphosphatemia: pharmacologic intervention yesterday, today and tomorrow. Clin Nephrol 2000;54:309. [PMID: 11076107]

Hypophosphatemia

- **Essentials of Diagnosis**
  - Serum phosphate < 2.5mg/dL; severe < 1.5 mg/dL
  - Generally asymptomatic with mild to moderate hypophosphatemia
  - Altered mental status, seizures, neuropathy, coma
  - Muscle weakness, rhabdomyolysis, hemolysis, impaired platelet and leukocyte function, respiratory failure, death in severe hypophosphatemia
  - Concurrent hypokalemia and hypomagnesemia
  - High risk groups: chronic alcoholics, diabetic ketoacidosis

- **Differential Diagnosis**
  - Chronic alcoholism
  - Refeeding after prolonged starvation
  - Diabetic ketoacidosis: insulin infusion, osmotic diuresis
  - Respiratory alkalosis
  - Hyperparathyroidism
  - Hypercalcemia
  - Vitamin D deficiency or malabsorption
  - Chronic ingestions of antacids, phosphate binders, or both
  - Postrenal transplantation

- **Treatment**
  - Oral phosphorus replacement preferred given fewer side effects
  - Intravenous phosphate may lead to metastatic calcification
  - Severe case with symptoms: intravenous phosphorous infusion given over 6 to 8 hours
  - Response to phosphorus replacement unpredictable; monitor levels during treatment
  - Replacement form with sodium or potassium salt; monitor these electrolytes as well
  - Prevention important in high risk groups
  - Address underlying etiology

- **Pearl**

In elderly patients with renal insufficiency, phosphate salts given for bowel preparation are associated with severe hyperphosphatemia, marked anion gap metabolic acidosis, and hypocalcemia.

Reference

DiMeglio LA et al: Disorders of phosphate metabolism. Endocrinol Metab Clin North Am 2000;29:591. [PMID: 11033762]

Hypervolemia

- **Essentials of Diagnosis**
  - Increase in extracellular volume: generalized or localized to certain compartments
  - Peripheral dependent pitting edema
  - Ascites with abdominal distention
  - Pulmonary edema or pleural effusions with dyspnea, rales, wheezes; resulting hypoxemia causing peripheral cyanosis, respiratory failure, altered mentation
  - Can be associated with decreased, normal or increased "effective" intravascular volume

- **Differential Diagnosis**
  - Congestive heart failure
  - Liver cirrhosis with ascites
  - Pre- and posthepatic portal hypertension with ascites
  - Nephrotic syndrome
  - Protein-losing enteropathy
  - Excess sodium intake: hypertonic solutions, dietary sources
  - Renal failure with oliguria
  - Hyperaldosteronism and hypercortisolism

- **Treatment**
  - Treatment depends on mechanism of disease
  - Diuretics mainstay of therapy
  - In reduced effective intravascular volume: delay diuresis until intravascular fluid deficit corrected; some worsening of hypervolemia acceptable during fluid resuscitation
  - Dietary sodium and fluid restriction
  - Large volume paracentesis or thoracentesis for symptom relief
  - Oxygen supplementation
  - Cardiogenic pulmonary edema: morphine, vasodilators (nitroprusside, hydralazine, ACE inhibitors), venodilators (nitrates), inotropes
  - Ventilatory support: mechanical or noninvasive ventilation
  - Hemodialysis or ultrafiltration in refractory cases

- **Pearl**

The common practice of renal-dose dopamine to induce diuresis has failed to be supported by the literature.

Reference

Kreimeier U: Pathophysiology of fluid imbalance. Crit Care 2000;4:S3. [PMID: 11255592]

Hypovolemia

- **Essentials of Diagnosis**
  - Reduced effective intravascular volume
  - Thirst, oliguria; may have altered mental status: confusion, lethargy, coma
  - Postural lightheadedness; orthostatic decrease in systolic blood pressure and increased heart rate
  - Hypotension, hypoperfusion, shock leading to hepatic, renal, cardiac dysfunction
  - Cold skin and extremities; dry axilla, sunken eyes some diagnostic value; poor skin turgor, dry mucous membranes poor diagnostic value
  - Reduced central venous pressure (CVP) and pulmonary capillary wedge pressure (PCWP)
  - Impaired renal function: BUN/creatinine > 30; reduced fractional excretion of sodium (FE_{Na}) $< 1\%$

- **Differential Diagnosis**
  - Gastrointestinal loss: vomiting, diarrhea, nasogastric suction, enteric fistulas
  - Renal loss: osmotic diuresis, diuretic use, post-ATN or obstructive diuresis
  - Skin loss: excessive sweating, burns
  - Hemorrhage: external or internal
  - Decreased intake of sodium and water
  - Adrenal insufficiency
  - Associated with increased extracellular volume: congestive heart failure, cirrhosis with ascites, hypoalbuminemia

- **Treatment**
  - Fluid resuscitation with colloid, crystalloid, or blood products
  - Amount of fluid depletion difficult to estimate; with known or suspected heart disease consider "fluid challenge"; follow urine output, CVP, PCWP, or blood pressure to guide therapy
  - Identify and correct source of volume loss
  - Careful review of daily intakes and outputs
  - Monitor for overcorrection and fluid overload states

- **Pearl**

Among all the physical findings for hypovolemia, an orthostatic increase in heart rate greater than 30 beats per minute has the highest specificity.

Reference

Boldt J: Volume therapy in the intensive care patient–we are still confused, but. . . Intensive Care Med 2000;26:1181. [PMID: 11089741]

Metabolic Acidosis

- ## Essentials of Diagnosis
  - Arterial pH < 7.35; decreased serum HCO_3^- and compensatory reduction in $Paco_2$; due to increased acid accumulation or decreased extracellular HCO_3^-
  - Fatigue, weakness, lethargy, somnolence, coma, nonspecific abdominal pain
  - Kussmaul (rapid and deep) respirations develop as acidosis progresses; rarely subjective dyspnea
  - Hypotension, shock poorly responsive to vasopressors; decreased cardiac contractility when pH < 7.10
  - Often associated with hyperkalemia
  - Calculate anion gap (AG) to help with diagnosis: $Na^+ - (HCO_3^- + Cl^-)$; normal value 12 ± 4 mEq/L
  - Calculate urinary anion gap with hyperchloremic nongap metabolic acidosis: urine $(Na^+ + K^+)$ − urine Cl^-; normal is < 0 due to presence of unmeasured ammonium cations; if > 0 then likely renal cause of metabolic acidosis

- ## Differential Diagnosis
  Anion gap acidosis (AG > 12)
  - Lactic acidosis   • Renal failure/uremia
  - Ketoacidosis: diabetic, ethanol induced, starvation
  - Toxin ingestion: salicylates, methanol, ethylene glycol, paraldehyde; not isopropyl alcohol
  - Massive rhabdomyolysis

  Non-anion-gap metabolic acidosis
  - Renal tubular acidosis (positive urinary anion gap); hypoaldosteronism, diarrhea

- ## Treatment
  - Identify and correct underlying disorder
  - Correct fluid and electrolyte disturbances
  - Bicarbonate therapy controversial in most cases of metabolic acidosis
  - Nonbicarbonate buffers (THAM, dichloroacetate, carbicarb) remain under investigation
  - Hemodialysis in severe, life-threatening circumstances
  - Mechanical ventilation to support respiratory failure

- ## Pearl
  An anion gap acidosis can exist even in the presence of a normal anion gap in the setting of hypoalbuminemia or pathological paraproteinemia. For every 1 g/dL reduction in serum albumin, a decrease of approximately 3 mmol in anion gap can be expected.

Reference

Gauthier PM et al: Metabolic acidosis in the intensive care unit. Crit Care Clin 2002;18:289. [PMID: 12053835]

Metabolic Alkalosis

- ■ Essentials of Diagnosis
  - Arterial pH > 7.45; increased serum HCO_3^- and compensatory elevation in $Paco_2$
  - Circumoral paresthesias, tetany, lethargy, confusion, seizure due to reduced ionized calcium
  - Hypoventilation usually not clinically evident
  - Often volume contracted with tachycardia and hypotension
  - If hypertension present consider glucocorticoid use, hyperaldosterone state; associated with hypokalemia
  - Lowers arrhythmia threshold; supraventricular and ventricular arrhythmias
  - Measure urinary chloride to differentiate between chloride-sensitive (volume-contracted) from chloride-resistant etiologies

- ■ Differential Diagnosis
  - Diuretics: loop, thiazides
  - Hypomagnesemia
  - Hypokalemia
  - Hyperaldosterone states
  - Posthypercapnic states
  - Cushing syndrome or disease
  - Hyper-renin states
  - Carbohydrate refeeding after starvation
  - Gastrointestinal loss: emesis, gastric suction, villous adenoma
  - Exogenous bicarbonate load: milk-alkali syndrome, citrate, lactate, acetate
  - Nonreabsorbed anions: penicillin, carbenicillin, ketones
  - Bartter or Gitelman syndrome

- ■ Treatment
  - Restore circulating volume with normal saline in chloride/saline-responsive states
  - In chloride/saline-resistant states, identify and address source of mineralocorticoid excess; spironolactone may play temporizing role in hyperaldosterone states
  - Correct electrolytes: magnesium, potassium
  - Acetazolamide used with extreme caution; administer only when volume status restored

- ■ Pearl

In a patient with borderline respiratory function, administration of acetazolamide in an attempt to "normalize" a metabolic alkalosis may precipitate fulminant respiratory failure due to increased production of carbon dioxide.

Reference

Khanna A et al: Metabolic alkalosis. Respir Care 2001;46:354. [PMID: 11262555]

Mixed Acid-Base Disorders

- **Essentials of Diagnosis**
  - Concurrent existence of more than one primary acid-base disturbance
  - Clues for mixed disorders: normal pH with abnormal $Paco_2$ and HCO_3^-; $Paco_2$ and HCO_3^- deviating in opposite directions; pH change in opposite direction for known primary disorder
  - Anion gap > 20 mmol/L always indicates primary metabolic acidosis
  - Obtain Δgap and "corrected" bicarbonate ($[HCO_3]_c$) to determine if additional metabolic process present: metabolic alkalosis if $[HCO_3]_c > 25$; nongap metabolic acidosis if $[HCO_3]_c < 25$
  - Check pH to determine if metabolic process primary (pH > 7.4 for metabolic alkalosis, pH < 7.4 for metabolic acidosis) or compensatory for respiratory process
  - Check $Paco_2$ for appropriate respiratory compensation for primary metabolic acidosis using $Paco_2 = 1.5 \times [HCO_3^-] + 8 \pm 2$; metabolic alkalosis using $\Delta Paco_2 = 2/3 \times \Delta HCO_3^-$

- **Differential Diagnosis**
  - Respiratory acidosis & metabolic acidosis: cardiopulmonary arrest, respiratory failure with renal failure
  - Respiratory alkalosis & metabolic alkalosis: cirrhosis with diuretic use or vomiting, pregnancy with hyperemesis, overventilation in COPD
  - Respiratory acidosis & metabolic alkalosis: COPD with diuretic use or vomiting
  - Respiratory alkalosis & metabolic acidosis: sepsis, salicylate intoxication, advanced liver disease with lactic acidosis
  - Metabolic acidosis & metabolic alkalosis: uremia or ketoacidosis with vomiting
  - Triple disturbance usually occurring in the setting of ketoacidosis with vomiting, liver disease, or sepsis

- **Treatment**
  - Identify and treat underlying etiology

- **Pearl**

Before embarking on excessive calculations to decipher any "complex acid-base disorder," always check for internal consistency between the pH, $Paco_2$, and serum HCO_3^- using the Henderson-Hasselbalch equation: $[H^-] = 24 \times (Paco_2/[HCO_3^-])$.

Reference

Kraut JA et al: Approach to patients with acid-base disorders. Respir Care 2001;46:392. [PMID: 11262558]

Respiratory Acidosis

- **Essentials of Diagnosis**
  - Arterial pH < 7.35; elevated $Paco_2$ and, if chronic, compensatory retention of serum HCO_3; due to ineffective alveolar ventilation or increased CO_2 production
  - Symptoms depend on absolute increase and rate of rise in $Paco_2$
  - Tremor, asterixis, incoordination, confusion, somnolence, coma
  - Headache, papilledema, retinal hemorrhages
  - Dyspnea, respiratory fatigue and failure
  - Hypoxemia common unless receiving supplemental oxygen

- **Differential Diagnosis**
  - Central nervous system depressants
  - Obesity hypoventilation syndrome
  - Chronic obstructive lung disease
  - Acute airway obstruction: acute aspiration, laryngospasm, bronchospasm
  - Restrictive defects: large pleural effusion, hemothorax, pneumothorax, fibrothorax, pulmonary fibrosis, flail chest
  - Pulmonary edema: cardiogenic or pulmonary permeability (ARDS)
  - Neurologic and neuromuscular disorders: Guillain-Barré syndrome, botulism, tetanus, phrenic nerve injury, cervical spine lesion, multiple sclerosis, poliomyelitis, myasthenia gravis
  - Organophosphate toxicity
  - Muscular weakness: electrolytes, muscular dystrophy

- **Treatment**
  - Correct underlying etiology
  - Avoid central suppressing agents
  - Mechanical ventilation or noninvasive positive-pressure ventilation
  - Aim to normalize pH and not $Paco_2$; overcorrection of chronic hypercapnia leads to alkalemia
  - Mild degree of respiratory acidosis well tolerated; may be beneficial in management of ARDS ("permissive hypercapnia")

- **Pearl**

The acute worsening of respiratory acidosis seen in chronic CO_2-retaining patients with COPD receiving high-flow oxygen supplementation is more likely due to worsening of $\dot{V}/\dot{Q}$ mismatch and not necessarily due to suppression of hypoxic drive.

Reference

Epstein SK et al: Respiratory acidosis. Respir Care 2001;46:366. [PMID: 11262556]

Respiratory Alkalosis

- **Essentials of Diagnosis**
    - Arterial pH > 7.45; decreased $Paco_2$ and compensatory reduction in serum HCO_3^-; due to increased and excessive alveolar ventilation
    - Decreased cerebral perfusion with confusion, lightheadedness, anxiety, irritability
    - Circumoral paresthesias, tetany, seizures; indistinguishable from hypocalcemia
    - Cardiac arrhythmias when pH > 7.6
    - Flattened ST segment or T-waves
    - Other clinical features associated with underlying etiology

- **Differential Diagnosis**
    - Meningoencephalitis
    - Pulmonary fibrosis
    - Pulmonary edema
    - Fever
    - Liver disease, hepatic failure
    - High altitude
    - Pregnancy and elevated progesterone states
    - Mechanical ventilation with overventilation
    - Central nervous system lesions: herniation, cerebrovascular accident
    - Hypoxemia
    - Pulmonary embolism
    - Anxiety, pain
    - Sepsis
    - Salicylate toxicity

- **Treatment**
    - Address and treat underlying disorders
    - Remove and avoid any central suppressing agents
    - Avoid excessive minute ventilation on mechanical ventilator
    - Increasing workload on ventilator (SIMV, CPAP, lengthening ventilator circuit tubing) to counteract primary respiratory alkalosis ineffective, dangerous, and not recommended
    - Paralysis with subsequent mechanical ventilation can be considered in severe cases

- **Pearl**

Primary hyperventilation must be distinguished from compensation for metabolic acidosis. The difference is that in respiratory alkalosis, low $Paco_2$ is primary and pH is above normal, whereas in metabolic acidosis pH is in the acidic range and low HCO_3^- represents the primary disturbance.

Reference

Foster GT: Respiratory alkalosis. Respir Care 2001;46:384.[PMID: 11262557]

Shock

Anaphylactic Shock

- **Essentials of Diagnosis**
  - Urticaria and angioedema; other manifestations include laryngeal edema, bronchospasm, pulmonary edema, tachycardia, hypotension, arrhythmias, abdominal cramps, diarrhea, syncope, seizures
  - Signs and symptoms typically develop within 5–30 minutes after exposure to offending agent; reaction can be delayed for several hours
  - Acute life-threatening immunologic reaction resulting from release of chemical mediators from mast cells and basophils
  - Classical IgE mediated agents include foods (peanuts, shellfish), medications, venoms, latex, vaccines, aspirin and NSAIDs, radiographic contrast media

- **Differential Diagnosis**
  - Vasovagal reactions
  - Pulmonary embolism
  - Myocardial ischemia
  - Septic or hypovolemic shock
  - Acute poisoning
  - Seizure disorder

- **Treatment**
  - Maintenance of airway, breathing, circulation with intubation, ventilatory support, volume expansion as needed
  - Epinephrine as soon as possible, 0.3–0.5 mg of 1:1000 dilution subcutaneously every 5–10 minutes as needed; use with caution in elderly and patients with coronary artery disease
  - Histamine antagonists such as diphenhydramine (H_1 antagonist) and ranitidine (H_2 antagonist)
  - Intravenous pressor agents such as dopamine may be required for persistent hypotension
  - Corticosteroids such as hydrocortisone may prevent late-phase manifestations which can occur up to 8 hours after initial presentation

- **Pearl**

Patients taking beta-blocking medications may be resistant to the effects of epinephrine. Atropine and glucagon may be helpful in these cases of anaphylactic shock.

Reference

Kemp SF et al: Anaphylaxis: a review of causes and mechanisms. J Allergy Clin Immunol 2002;110:341. [PMID: 12209078]

Cardiac Compressive Shock

- **Essentials of Diagnosis**
  - Low cardiac output state caused by compression of heart or great vessels
  - Hypotension, tachycardia, cool extremities, elevated neck veins, pulsus paradoxus, distant heart sounds, oliguria, altered mental status
  - ECG with reduced amplitudes; may have electrical alternans
  - "Water bottle" shaped cardiac silhouette on chest radiograph
  - Echocardiogram demonstrates fluid within pericardium causing right cardiac chamber collapse
  - Pulmonary artery catheter reveals equalization of central venous, pulmonary capillary, and pulmonary artery diastolic pressures with low cardiac index
  - Cardiac tamponade most common cause; accumulation of fluid in pericardial sac sufficient to prevent filling of cardiac chambers
  - Causes of cardiac tamponade: malignancy, trauma, uremia, connective tissue disorders, uremia, infection, idiopathic pericarditis

- **Differential Diagnosis**
  - Restrictive cardiomyopathy
  - Right ventricular infarction
  - Left ventricular failure
  - Constrictive pericarditis
  - Tension pneumothorax

- **Treatment**
  - Intravascular volume expansion with intravenous fluids
  - Immediate drainage of pericardial effusion via pericardiocentesis
  - Pericardial catheter can be left in place for period of days for ongoing drainage
  - Surgical or percutaneous balloon pericardial window can be performed for definitive treatment depending on cause of effusion and rapidity of reaccumulation

- **Pearl**

The cardinal finding of elevated neck veins in cardiac tamponade may be absent in the volume depleted patient.

Reference

Bogolioubov A et al: Circulatory shock. Crit Care Clin 2001;17:697. [PMID: 11525054]

Cardiogenic Shock

■ Essentials of Diagnosis
- Severely low cardiac output state caused by myocardial or valvular dysfunction leading to inadequate tissue perfusion
- Hypotension, cool extremities, distended neck veins, third heart sound, oliguria, respiratory distress due to pulmonary edema
- Pulmonary artery catheter typically demonstrates elevated central venous pressure, increased pulmonary capillary wedge pressure, high systemic vascular resistance, low cardiac index (< 2 L/min/m^2)
- Acute myocardial infarction most common cause
- Other etiologies: acute valvular abnormalities, septal defects or rupture, free wall rupture, traumatic myocardial contusion

■ Differential Diagnosis
- Hypovolemic shock
- Aortic dissection
- Septic shock
- Severe aortic stenosis

■ Treatment
- When cardiogenic shock results from acute myocardial infarction, efforts to improve myocardial perfusion and reduce ischemia are priority; consider prompt thrombolytic therapy or cardiac catheterization with primary coronary intervention
- Intravascular volume should be optimized; pulmonary artery catheter may help; goal pulmonary capillary wedge pressure 17–18 mm Hg
- Dobutamine useful in congestive heart failure and cardiogenic shock given its positive inotropic effects, minimal chronotropic and peripheral vasoconstricting properties
- Dopamine or norepinephrine for persistent hypotension
- Vasodilators such as nitroglycerin and nitroprusside can lower left ventricular afterload; use often limited by hypotension
- Diuretics helpful in treatment of pulmonary edema
- Intra-aortic balloon pump can be utilized for refractory hypotension with poor organ perfusion

■ Pearl

In patients with acute myocardial infarction, the onset of cardiogenic shock is often delayed, with median onset of shock occurring 5.5–7 hours after the initial ischemic insult.

Reference

Hollenberg SM: Cardiogenic shock. Crit Care Clin 2001;17:391. [PMID: 11450323]

Hypovolemic Shock

- **Essentials of Diagnosis**
  - Hypotension, cool extremities, collapsed neck veins, poor capillary refill
  - Orthostatic hypotension and oliguria
  - Elevated BUN to creatinine ratio, concentrated hematocrit; anemia if blood loss is cause
  - Rapid correction of signs occurs with adequate fluid resuscitation
  - Trauma most common cause
  - Other etiologies: gastrointestinal bleeding, fistulas, diarrhea, excessive diuresis, diabetes insipidus, burns, disruption of suture lines

- **Differential Diagnosis**
  - Cardiogenic shock
  - Septic Shock
  - Neurogenic shock
  - Anaphylactic shock

- **Treatment**
  - Establish intravenous access with two large bore catheters
  - Rapid fluid resuscitation; infuse at rate adequate to correct calculated or estimated fluid deficit
  - Fluid for resuscitation can be crystalloid (normal saline, lactated Ringer's), colloid (albumin, hetastarch, dextran), blood products (packed red blood cells, plasma)
  - Transfusion of platelets and coagulation factors may be necessary if large volume of packed red blood cells given
  - Continue rapid fluid resuscitation until reversal of abnormal signs such as improved blood pressure, decreased heart rate, increased urine output; avoid excessive volume leading to pulmonary edema
  - Evaluate patient for source of blood loss to tailor additional therapeutic interventions

- **Pearl**

If oliguria is not present in the face of clinical hypovolemic shock, evaluate the urine for the presence of osmotically active substances such as glucose, radiographic dyes, or toxins

Reference

Orlinsky M et al: Current controversies in shock and resuscitation. Surg Clin North Am 2001;81:1217. [PMID: 11766174]

Neurogenic Shock

- **Essentials of Diagnosis**
  - Loss of peripheral vasomotor tone as a result of spinal cord injury, regional anesthesia, autonomic blocking agents
  - Signs and symptoms depend on location within nervous system
  - Injury above midthorax/T6 level: hypotension and bradycardia from loss of thoracic sympathetic tone, vasodilatation, increased vagal tone
  - Spinal cord interruption below the midthorax/T6 level: activation of adrenergic system above level of injury leading to tachycardia and increased cardiac contractility
  - Extremities are warm above and cool below level of injury
  - Hypotension may be profound
  - Decreased venous return and cardiac output due to peripheral venous blood pooling
  - Cervical, thoracic, and/or lumbosacral spine imaging to evaluate for fractures; MRI and CT scan for further evaluation of spinal cord

- **Differential Diagnosis**
  - Anaphylactic shock
  - Hypovolemic shock

- **Treatment**
  - Endotracheal intubation, ventilatory support, volume resuscitation, vasopressors as needed
  - Blood pressure may improve with adequate fluid resuscitation
  - Fiberoptic or nasal intubation may be required if cervical spine instability suspected
  - Norepinephrine or phenylephrine for hypotension refractory to fluids

- **Pearl**

Isolated head trauma does not cause neurogenic shock but can cause the Cushing reflex of increased blood pressure accompanied by bradycardia.

Reference

Manley G et al: Hypotension, hypoxia, and head injury: frequency, duration, and consequences. Arch Surg 2001;136:1118. [PMID: 11585502]

Septic Shock

- **Essentials of Diagnosis**
  - Hypotension and inadequate organ perfusion despite adequate fluid resuscitation in presence of systemic inflammatory response syndrome (SIRS) due to infection
  - Wide spectrum of clinical findings ranging from subtle fever, tachycardia, tachypnea to severe shock with multisystem organ failure
  - Warm skin with vasodilated peripheral vascular bed
  - Associated organ system dysfunction: lactic acidosis, acute respiratory distress syndrome (ARDS), acute renal failure, disseminated intravascular coagulopathy (DIC), central nervous system dysfunction, hepatobiliary abnormalities
  - Elevated cardiac output, low systemic vascular resistance, low blood pressure, elevated pulse pressure

- **Differential Diagnosis**
  - Hypovolemic shock
  - Neurogenic shock
  - Cardiogenic shock
  - Anaphylactic shock

- **Treatment**
  - Antibiotics directed against likely sources of infection instituted as quickly as possible; initial regimen often empiric as causative microorganism rarely known initially
  - Aggressive fluid resuscitation with blood products, crystalloid, or colloid; central venous pressure monitoring may be helpful
  - Vasopressors (dopamine or norepinephrine) if hypotension persists after initial fluid resuscitation
  - Ventilatory support to maintain adequate oxygenation and ventilation
  - Low-dose hydrocortisone (50 mg every 6 hours) when evidence of adrenal insufficiency complicates sepsis
  - Adjunctive recombinant human activated protein C demonstrated statistically significant decrease in mortality in appropriate patients with severe sepsis and multiorgan system dysfunction

- **Pearl**

Elderly and debilitated patients may not exhibit significant symptoms at the onset of sepsis.

Reference

Hotchkiss RS: The pathophysiology and treatment of sepsis. N Engl J Med 2003;348:138. [PMID: 12519925]

7

Pulmonary Disease

Acute Chest Syndrome in Sickle Cell Anemia

- **Essentials of Diagnosis**
  - New pulmonary infiltrates, fever, chest pain, cough, sputum production, dyspnea in patient with sickle cell disease (SCD)
  - May appear toxic with high fever, tachypnea, tachycardia
  - Rales, wheezes, decreased breath sounds, dullness to percussion
  - Chest radiographs most commonly reveal lower lobe infiltrates, atelectasis
  - Anemia, thrombocytopenia, leukocytosis, indirect hyperbilirubinemia, elevated LDH
  - Often develops after vaso-occlusive crisis
  - Etiology multifactorial but clinically resembles pneumonia
  - Respiratory distress related to infection, pulmonary fat embolism from bone infarct, pulmonary vascular occlusion by sickled erythrocytes, iatrogenic fluid overload, hypoxemia, splinting due to painful rib or sternal infarcts
  - Risk factors: children, hemoglobin SS genotype, low hemoglobin F, elevated WBC, previous acute chest syndrome
  - Most common cause of death and second most common cause of hospitalization in adults with sickle cell anemia

- **Differential Diagnosis**
  - Pulmonary embolism
  - Community acquired pneumonia
  - Sickle cell pain crisis
  - Congestive heart failure
  - Myocardial infarction
  - ARDS

- **Treatment**
  - Supportive care with oxygen, bronchodilators, incentive spirometry, pain control
  - Empiric antibiotics to cover community-acquired pneumonia; include chlamydia and mycoplasma coverage
  - Fluid management individualized to avoid pulmonary edema
  - Role of blood transfusion unclear but exchange transfusion with goal to reduce hemoglobin S to 20–30% indicated for persistent hypoxemia and tachypnea, deteriorating vital signs

- **Pearl**

More than 50% of patients present with an acute pain crisis 2.5 days prior to the onset of findings consistent with acute chest syndrome.

Reference

Platt O: The acute chest syndrome of sickle cell disease. N Engl J Med 2000;342:1904. [PMID: 10861328]

Acute Inhalation Injury

- **Essentials of Diagnosis**
  - Suspect in patients with facial burns, singed facial hair, intra-oral burns, carbonaceous deposits in oropharynx
  - Findings depend on exposure: transient airway irritation; bronchospasm; pulmonary edema; toxic pneumonitis with fever, chills, chest pain; flu-like syndrome with cough, myalgias, fatigue; respiratory failure
  - Edema, erythema, mucosal ulcerations, carbonaceous material on laryngoscopy
  - Injury sustained is function of toxins and their physical properties, intensity and duration of exposure, host factors
  - Water solubility determines where inhaled gas gets deposited; highly soluble gases (ammonia, sulfur dioxide, hydrogen chloride) cause acute irritant injury to eyes, nose, upper airway; spare lower airways; less soluble gases (phosgene, ozone, nitrogen oxides) penetrate and damage lower airways
  - Most particles <100 microns enter airways; <10 microns enter lower airways; <5 microns deposit in terminal bronchioles and alveoli
  - Direct thermal injury occurs from steam exposure overwhelming protective cooling defenses
  - Obtain carboxyhemoglobin level in all smoke inhalations
  - Elevated lactate may indicate cyanide toxicity
  - Poor prognostic signs: rales, burns to face, hypoxemia, altered mental status, respiratory compromise

- **Differential Diagnosis**
  - Asthma or COPD exacerbation
  - Cardiogenic pulmonary edema
  - ARDS
  - Pneumonia

- **Treatment**
  - Supplemental oxygen; important in treating CO poisoning
  - Early intubation if signs of upper airway compromise
  - Pulmonary toilet with bronchodilators and inspiratory maneuvers; antibiotics if clinical signs of pneumonia develop
  - Steroid therapy remains controversial
  - Treat for cyanide toxicity if suspected

- **Pearl**

A detailed exposure history may alert the clinician to the possibility of delayed effects and later clinical deterioration.

Reference

Rabinowitz PM et al: Acute inhalation injury. Clin Chest Med 2002;23:707. [PMID: 12512160]

Anaphylaxis

- **Essentials of Diagnosis**
  - Urticaria, pruritis, flushing, shortness of breath, localized edema; onset 5–60 minutes after exposure to inciting antigen
  - Wheezing, laryngeal edema, respiratory failure, pulmonary edema
  - Hypotension (anaphylactic shock)
  - Causes in ICU: antibiotics (penicillins), radiocontrast media, food, blood products; rarely to latex or other allergens
  - Antigen exposure through air, contact, blood or other injection with immediate, life-threatening allergic reaction; usually IgE mediated immediate hypersensitivity; may be non-antibody-mediated
  - Release of histamine, complement components, prostaglandins, and leukotrienes from mast cells and basophils through bound IgE
  - May or may not have history of previous anaphylaxis

- **Differential Diagnosis**
  - Angioedema
  - Asthma
  - Urticaria
  - Vasculitis

- **Treatment**
  - Maintain airway and cardiopulmonary function; endotracheal intubation
  - Remove antigen; discontinue drug or blood products
  - Epinephrine, 0.5–1.0 mL of 1:10,000 IV for severe airway compromise or shock; otherwise 0.3–0.5 mL of 1:1000 subcutaneously
  - Hydrocortisone, 100 mg every 6–8 hours
  - Diphenhydramine, 25–50 mg IV every 4–6 hours plus cimetidine, 300 mg IV every 8–12 hours
  - May require large volumes of IV crystalloids (0.9% NaCl); epinephrine, dopamine for persistent hypotension
  - Observe for late or persistent reactions

- **Pearl**

Radiocontrast agents are the most common cause of anaphylaxis in the ICU.

Reference

Kemp SF et al: Anaphylaxis: a review of causes and mechanisms. J Allergy Clin Immunol 2002; 110:341 [PMID: 12209078]

Angioedema

- ■ **Essentials of Diagnosis**
  - Acute or chronic recurrent episodes of facial, cutaneous, mucosal membrane swelling; may have narrowing of upper airways
  - May be associated with urticaria
  - Acute related to medications (angiotensin converting enzyme (ACE) inhibitors), NSAIDs, aspirin
  - Chronic congenital (autosomal dominant C1 esterase inhibitor deficiency), rarely acquired chronic angioedema
  - Mechanisms similar to anaphylaxis but different mediators and precipitating events
  - Associated conditions include malignancy, collagen vascular disease, infections, allergic phenomena

- ■ **Differential Diagnosis**
  - Anaphylaxis
  - Acute asthma exacerbation
  - Upper airway obstruction including acute epiglottis, foreign body, retropharyngeal abscess
  - Allergic transfusion reactions

- ■ **Treatment**
  - Maintain patent airway
  - Assess severity; anticipate further complications
  - Discontinue suspected drugs especially ACE inhibitors
  - Administer epinephrine, antihistamines, corticosteroids as for anaphylaxis
  - Long-term therapy for hereditary angioedema may include recombinant C1 inhibitor concentrate, fresh frozen plasma, danazol

- ■ **Pearl**

Angioedema from angiotensin-converting enzyme inhibitors can occur anytime after the drug is started, even after years without side effects; now also reported with angiotensin-receptor blockers as well.

Reference

Cohen EG et al: Changing trends in angioedema. Ann Otol Rhinol Laryngol 2001;110:701. [PMID: 11510724]

Chest Tube Thoracostomy

■ Essential Concepts

- Bedside procedure performed to remove fluid or air from pleural space or to instill agents to ablate pleural space
- May require ultrasound or CT imaging to guide tube placement if loculated fluid or air collection
- No absolute contraindication exists but care should be taken in patients with coagulopathies, bullae, large effusions due to main airway occlusion, previous thoracotomy, pleurodesis

■ Essentials of Management

- Chest tube size depends on type of material to be aspirated: smaller caliber tubes (12 to 28 Fr) for air and larger tubes for fluid (32 to 36 Fr for effusion, 36 to 42 Fr for pus or blood)
- Drainage system prepared at bedside before beginning procedure: three "bottle" system consisting of collection compartment, water seal chamber, manometer for suction control
- Most chest tubes inserted in fourth or fifth intercostal space along anterior axillary line
- Positioning of tube depends on indication for insertion: apically placed tubes for pneumothoraces; dependently placed tubes for pleural effusions or fluid drainage
- Once tube inserted into pleural space, apply suction (10–20 cm H_2O) until all air or fluid removed
- System should be evaluated to assure proper function: fluctuation of fluid column with respiration suggests tube is within pleural space and subjected to intrapleural pressures
- Once lung fully expanded, air leak resolved, or drainage < 150 mL per day, system can be switched to water seal and monitored; if lung remains expanded and no significant reaccumulation of fluid or air, tube can be removed
- If persistent air leak, evaluate entire system to locate source as it may come from within apparatus and not patient
- If drainage ceases, "milking" tubing may help reestablish flow
- Complications: improper positioning, subcutaneous emphysema, bleeding, intercostal nerve damage, diaphragm or abdominal organ injury, pain, re-expansion pulmonary edema

■ Pearl

A tension pneumothorax may develop if a chest tube is clamped during transportation or movement of the patient.

Reference

Gilbert TB et al: Chest tubes: indications, placement, management, and complications. J Intensive Care Med 1993;8:73. [PMID: 10148363]

Obesity-Hypoventilation Syndrome

■ Essentials of Diagnosis
- Lethargy and coma from acute respiratory acidosis or signs of right heart failure (weight gain, lower extremity edema)
- Dyspnea or wheezing suggests presence of concomitant obstructive lung disease or pulmonary edema
- Hypercapnic respiratory failure due to combination of depressed ventilatory responsiveness to carbon dioxide (CO_2) and hypoxemia, increased work of breathing, possible abnormal heart and lung function
- Uncommon condition affecting morbidly obese individuals
- Often develop pulmonary hypertension leading to cor pulmonale
- Variable relationship to obstructive sleep apnea

■ Differential Diagnosis
- Central nervous system disease
- Cardiomyopathy
- Hypothyroidism and myxedema coma
- Central respiratory drive suppressants: benzodiazepines, opioids

■ Treatment
- Ventilatory support with mechanical ventilation may be necessary to provide adequate oxygen and to improve ventilatory drive by resetting hypercapnic central drive sensitivity
- Consider noninvasive positive pressure ventilation; especially if concomitant obstructive sleep apnea present
- Diuresis with oxygen and diuretics may help volume overload
- Assess for presence of abnormal left ventricular function that may require additional treatment with afterload reduction and beta-blockers
- Medroxyprogesterone acetate may be beneficial for long-term management but role in acute decompensation unclear
- Use of sedative-hypnotic and centrally suppressing agents contraindicated

■ Pearl
Patients with obesity-hypoventilation syndrome who present with respiratory failure will often regain significant ventilatory responsiveness to CO_2 after several days of mechanical ventilatory support.

Reference

Krachman S et al: Hypoventilation syndromes. Clin Chest Med 1998;19:139. [PMID: 9554224]

Obstructive Sleep Apnea Syndrome

- ■ Essentials of Diagnosis
  - Excessive daytime somnolence with evidence of upper airway obstruction occurring at any site above glottis during sleep
  - Obstructive events last 10–90 seconds and terminate with arousal from sleep leading to sleep fragmentation
  - Accessory muscle use, intercostal retractions, paradoxical inspiratory chest wall movements observed during apneas
  - Acute hypercapnia, hypoxemia, disrupted sleep, hemodynamic alterations occur with obstruction and can lead to systemic hypertension and cor pulmonale
  - Bradycardia with pauses up to 13 seconds and ventricular ectopy seen in severe cases during desaturations
  - Daytime hypoventilation not common
  - Common characteristics: male sex, age over 40 years, habitual snoring, observed apneas, systemic hypertension
  - Risk factors: obesity, tonsillar hypertrophy, craniofacial abnormalities with narrowing of posterior oropharynx, edema of airway structures, diminished neural reflexes or ventilatory control

- ■ Differential Diagnosis
  - Simple snoring
  - Cheyne-Stokes respirations
  - Central sleep apnea syndrome

- ■ Treatment
  - Nasal continuous positive airway pressure (CPAP) is treatment of choice; acts as pneumatic splint preventing airway closure
  - Oxygen therapy alone can prolong apneic events and should be used with careful monitoring
  - Endotracheal intubation or tracheostomy highly effective for select patients failing noninvasive ventilation
  - Lateral decubitus position or elevated head of bed preferred
  - Use of sedative-hypnotic and centrally suppressing agents contraindicated
  - No role for respiratory stimulants or carbonic anhydrase inhibitors

- ■ Pearl

Obstructive sleep apnea syndrome should be suspected in obese hypersomnolent snorers who are hypertensive.

Reference

Strollo PJ Jr: Indications for treatment of obstructive sleep apnea in adults. Clin Chest Med 2003;24:307. [PMID: 12800786]

Pleural Effusions in the ICU

- **Essentials of Diagnosis**
  - Accumulation of fluid within pleural space
  - Symptoms range from none to dyspnea, pleuritic chest pain, respiratory failure
  - Radiographic findings may be subtle in ICU patients as radiographs frequently taken with patient in semirecumbent or reclining position; < 500 mL of fluid may appear as haziness over lower lung fields in these positions
  - Primary pleural disease rarely reason for admission to ICU; pleura can be secondarily affected as part of spectrum of critical illness
  - Clinical relevance of small effusions (< 100 mL) found only by ultrasound or CT scan in this patient population remains unclear
  - Performing thoracentesis generally safe in critically ill patients
  - Risk factors for development of pleural effusion in ICU include immobility, sedation, paralytic agents
  - Common etiologies: congestive heart failure (bilateral transudates or "pseudoexudate"), atelectasis (unilateral transudate), uncomplicated parapneumonic effusion (unilateral exudate)

- **Differential Diagnosis**
  - Parenchymal consolidation or atelectasis
  - Pleural thickening
  - Lung or pleural-based mass
  - Elevated hemidiaphragm

- **Treatment**
  - Diagnostic thoracentesis if pleural effusion and fever, lack of clinical response to antibiotic therapy, atypical presentation for underlying disease
  - Majority resolve with therapy aimed at underlying disease
  - Antibiotic therapy alone for uncomplicated parapneumonic effusions; chest tube thoracostomy for empyemas
  - Chest tube drainage for complicated parapneumonic effusions, large hemothoraces, symptomatic malignant effusions

- **Pearl**

Consider thoracentesis in critically ill patients with pleural effusions as the finding of an unsuspected infectious etiology will have a dramatic impact on therapy and outcome.

Reference

Fartoukh M et al: Clinically documented pleural effusions in medical ICU patients. Chest 2002;121:178. [PMID:11796448]

Pneumothorax

- **Essentials of Diagnosis**
  - Shortness of breath, chest pain, hypoxemia, hypercapnia; chest resonant to percussion, asymmetric decreased breath sounds
  - If tension pneumothorax (check-valve mechanism causing positive intrapleural pressure), hypotension, cardiopulmonary arrest
  - Air collects in pleural space (or extrapleural space between parietal pleura and chest wall) from lung rupture or disruption of chest wall; subsequent lung collapse
  - Etiologies include: spontaneous; traumatic; complication of lung abscess, *Pneumocystis carinii*, tuberculosis, emphysema; complication of mechanical ventilation, thoracentesis, central venous catheter, pleural or lung biopsy
  - Chest radiograph: separation of lung from chest wall, deep sulcus sign (hyperlucent costophrenic angle); pneumomediastinum; subcutaneous air in neck or chest wall

- **Differential Diagnosis**
  - Atelectasis
  - Pleural effusion
  - Pulmonary embolism
  - Upper or central airway obstruction

- **Treatment**
  - High F_{IO_2} speeds resolution
  - Observation only if small pneumothorax in stable patient due to inadvertent introduction of air (thoracentesis), no further accumulation, not on mechanical ventilation
  - Otherwise evacuate air with percutaneous catheter if moderate size, no mechanical ventilation, stable; surgical tube thoracostomy for all others
  - Emergent evacuation by catheter or chest tube if hypotension, respiratory failure
  - Attach pleural drain to collection device with "water seal" and suction; when no air leak, discontinue suction; if lung remains inflated, consider removing tube

- **Pearl**

If a pneumothorax is suspected and a chest radiograph with the patient in a supine position does not demonstrate a pneumothorax, a CT scan (which is very sensitive) should be obtained.

Reference

Chen KY et al: Pneumothorax in the ICU: patient outcomes and prognostic factors. Chest 2002;122:678. [PMID: 12171850]

Pulmonary Thromboembolism

- ■ Essentials of Diagnosis
    - • Dyspnea, tachypnea, tachycardia, pleuritic chest pain; calf pain and swelling consistent with deep vein thrombosis (DVT)
    - • Hypotension, syncope, cyanosis, shock if "massive" (>50% pulmonary vascular bed occlusion); or submassive in patient with poor cardiopulmonary reserve
    - • Mild to moderate hypoxemia, increased $P(A\text{-}a)O_2$, mildly reduced Pa_{CO_2}
    - • Sinus tachycardia most frequent ECG abnormality; "S1Q3T3" pattern of right heart strain considered highly predictive but seen in <12% of patients with pulmonary embolism (PE)
    - • D-dimer, fibrin degradation product in patients with DVT and PE usually >500 μg/dL
    - • Normal chest radiograph in hypoxemic individual should lead to suspicion of PE; other common radiographic findings include platelike atelectasis, small pleural effusions
    - • Diagnostic imaging techniques include Doppler ultrasound of symptomatic extremity, radionuclide ventilation-perfusion scan, helical (spiral) CT angiogram, pulmonary angiogram
    - • Risk factors: immobilization, trauma to extremity, previous DVT/PE, recent surgery, obesity, nephrotic syndrome, congestive heart failure, stroke, malignancy, estrogen use

- ■ Differential Diagnosis
    - • Acute coronary syndrome
    - • Acute chest syndrome
    - • Spontaneous pneumothorax
    - • Fat embolism
    - • Asthma

- ■ Treatment
    - • Prevention in ICU patients with risk factors is paramount
    - • If no contraindications, once DVT or PE suspected, anticoagulation with unfractionated or low-molecular-weight heparin should be instituted while awaiting confirmatory diagnostic testing
    - • Thrombolytic therapy may be option in patients with "massive PE"; may consider in patients with hypotension to hasten hemodynamic stabilization

- ■ Pearl

Ventilation-perfusion scans in patients with COPD are generally considered to be of limited value because airway obstruction can cause a falsely positive perfusion defect due to hypoxemic mediated vasoconstriction.

Reference

Rocha AT, et al: Venous thromboembolism in intensive care patients. Clin Chest Med 2003;24:103. [PMID: 12685059]

8

Respiratory Failure

Acute Respiratory Distress Syndrome (ARDS)

- ■ Essentials of Diagnosis
  - • Severe hypoxemia refractory to supplemental oxygen ($Pa_{O_2}/F_{IO_2} < 200–300$); acute diffuse chest radiograph infiltrates consistent with noncardiogenic pulmonary edema (increased lung permeability); no evidence of heart failure; if measured, normal or low pulmonary artery wedge pressure
  - • 75–80% due to sepsis, pneumonia, aspiration of gastric contents, severe trauma; other causes: fat embolism, pancreatitis, transfusion related lung injury, amniotic fluid embolism
  - • Mortality 30–60%; highest in sepsis, elderly, multiorgan system failure; due to nonrespiratory organ failure, infection; rarely respiratory failure

- ■ Differential Diagnosis
  - • Cardiogenic pulmonary edema
  - • Severe extrapulmonary right-to-left shunt (intracardiac shunt)
  - • Severe localized pneumonia or atelectasis without diffuse lung involvement

- ■ Treatment
  - • Treat underlying disease (sepsis, trauma, pneumonia, pancreatitis)
  - • High oxygen concentrations ($F_{IO_2} > 0.4$)
  - • Endotracheal intubation, mechanical ventilation needed for increased work of breathing
  - • Positive end-expiratory pressure
  - • Low tidal volume (<6 mL/kg) improves survival; may lead to hypercapnia (keep f < 35/min)
  - • Minimal fluid intake and diuretics may help reduce pulmonary edema; may not be compatible with treating underlying diseases
  - • Complications of high F_{IO_2}: lung injury; high positive end-expiratory pressure (PEEP): low cardiac output, hypotension, pneumothorax, lung injury

- ■ Pearl

Attack rate of ARDS for patients with similar underlying disorders may be higher in chronic alcoholics, smokers, and the elderly.

Reference

Ware LB et al: The acute respiratory distress syndrome. N Engl J Med 2000;342:1334. [PMID: 10793167]

Air Embolism Syndrome

- **Essentials of Diagnosis**
  - Sudden cardiovascular collapse with hypotension, hypoxemia, respiratory distress, occasionally stroke symptoms and signs caused by air entering systemic venous, pulmonary arterial, pulmonary venous circulation
  - In ICU, most frequently related to central venous catheter insertion, removal, disconnection, or accidental injection of air
  - Seen in trauma, diving accidents, hemodialysis, open heart surgery, thoracotomy, neurosurgical procedures
  - May have paradoxical arterial emboli with stroke or systemic arterial occlusion via patent foramen ovale or pulmonary right-to-left shunts
  - Air bubbles occasionally seen on chest imaging, echocardiogram, head CT scan

- **Differential Diagnosis**
  - Shock: cardiogenic, hypovolemic, anaphylactic
  - Pulmonary thromboembolism
  - Cardiac tamponade
  - Tension pneumothorax

- **Treatment**
  - Place patient on left side, head down
  - If air entry from CVP catheter, stop air entry; aspirate air from right ventricle
  - Supportive care, oxygen, cardiopulmonary resuscitation
  - Hyperbaric oxygen recommended but usually impractical and delayed
  - Prevention: place CVP catheter with patient head down, prevent air injection, remove catheter with patient head down, take precautions to avoid accidental disconnection

- **Pearl**

Position patient to keep central venous catheter entry site below "heart" level whenever inserting, adjusting, using, or removing the catheter.

Reference

Heckmann JG et al: Neurologic manifestations of cerebral air embolism as a complication of central venous catheterization. Crit Care Med 2000;28:1621. [PMID: 10834723]

Aspiration Pneumonitis & Pneumonia

- ■ Essentials of Diagnosis
  - • Aspiration pneumonitis: chemical irritation (food, gastric acid) plus inflammation; may be witnessed; symptoms and chest radiograph changes 2–5 hours after event; aspiration of gastric contents from impaired consciousness, loss of gag reflex, enteral feeding, impaired gastric motility, endotracheal intubation, supine positioning
  - • Aspiration pneumonia: aspiration of bacteria from oropharynx or stomach; usually unwitnessed; increased with periodontal infection, alcoholism, impaired consciousness; increased in critically ill (altered bacterial flora, impaired swallowing, endotracheal intubation, advanced age)

- ■ Differential Diagnosis
  - • Community-acquired pneumonia, tuberculosis, fungal pneumonia
  - • Ventilator-associated pneumonia
  - • Pulmonary edema

- ■ Treatment
  - • Treat respiratory failure due to acute lung injury
  - • Keep airway clear by suctioning; may need endotracheal intubation if severe
  - • Antibiotics not needed in pneumonitis unless high risk of bacterial colonization of stomach (small bowel obstruction, inhibition of gastric acid production) or fever, abnormal chest radiograph, respiratory failure > 48 hours after suspected aspiration; corticosteroids contraindicated
  - • Aspiration pneumonia: Antibiotics indicated; if hospitalized < 72 hours, treat as community-acquired pneumonia (ceftriaxone or levofloxacin); hospitalized > 72 hours or resident in long-term care facility, treat Gram-negative bacilli including Pseudomonas; high likelihood of anaerobic or mixed infection (alcoholism, periodontal disease), levofloxacin or ceftriaxone plus clindamycin or metronidazole

- ■ Pearl

Routine elevation of head of bed to 30–45 degrees decreases risk of aspiration and ventilator-associated pneumonia by as much as 60% over first 7 days.

Reference

Marik PE: Aspiration pneumonitis and aspiration pneumonia. N Engl J Med 2001;344:665. [PMID: 11228282]

Life-Threatening Hemoptysis

- **■ Essentials of Diagnosis**
  - Hemoptysis with large volume in patient with normal pulmonary function, or smaller volumes if impaired cardiopulmonary function, cough, consciousness
  - Tuberculosis, tuberculous cavity with aspergilloma (mycetoma), trauma, mitral stenosis; less common with lung cancer
  - > 600 mL hemoptysis in 16 hours has 75% mortality without surgery; < 600 mL about 5% mortality
  - Respiratory failure occurs before hemodynamic compromise with hemoptysis
  - Risk factors: coagulopathy, infection, thrombocytopenia, renal failure
  - Bronchial arteries source 90%, pulmonary arteries 10%

- **■ Differential Diagnosis**
  - Severe epistaxis
  - Upper gastrointestinal bleeding

- **■ Treatment**
  - Establish and maintain patent airway
  - Consider endotracheal intubation if cough inadequate; double-lumen split bronchial intubation useful, but requires experienced personnel to position
  - Measure quantity of blood expectorated over time
  - Establish severity of underlying lung disease (chest radiograph, CT scan, arterial blood gases)
  - Localize bleeding site with fiberoptic bronchoscopy (if mild to moderate bleeding) or bronchial arteriography
  - Control bleeding; bronchial artery embolization preferred over emergent surgical resection
  - Definitive therapy requires surgery but outcome better if delayed
  - Treat underlying infection (bacterial, tuberculous), correct thrombocytopenia or coagulopathy

- **■ Pearl**

Don't worry about the patient's loss of blood; if there is that much hemoptysis, the patient will asphyxiate first.

Reference

Jean-Baptiste E: Clinical assessment and management of massive hemoptysis. Crit Care Med 2000;28:1642. [PMID: 10834728]

Mechanical Ventilation

■ Essential Concepts

- Usually delivered through endotracheal tube; sometimes "noninvasively" using mask (noninvasive positive-pressure ventilation or NIPPV)
- Defined by changeover from expiration to inspiration ("trigger"); and changeover from inspiration to expiration ("mode")
- Volume-Cycle Ventilation (VCV): most common; preset tidal volume (V_T) each breath; preset breaths per minute or patient may "trigger" at own rate; preset inspiratory flow rate or time
- Pressure-Controlled Ventilation (PCV): inspired flow at preset pressure; V_T determined by pressure, compliance of respiratory system; preset breaths per minute or patient may "trigger"; set inspiratory time
- Pressure-Support Ventilation (PSV): provides preset inspiratory pressure but V_T determined by patient effort and pressure gradient between ventilator and patient; used mostly for weaning
- Intermittent Mandatory Ventilation (IMV): provides preset breaths per minute; patient can breathe spontaneously (with or without PSV) at other times; used mostly for weaning
- May cause impaired venous return leading to hypotension, low cardiac output; pneumothorax, pneumomediastinum, lung injury
- Indications: respiratory failure, especially worsening gas exchange or muscle fatigue; absent (apnea) or inadequate ventilatory drive; high work of breathing; hemodynamic instability or acute pulmonary edema

■ Essentials of Management

- Select ventilator mode (VCV, PCV, PSV, IMV)
- For VCV or IMV: preset V_T, backup rate, peak inspiratory flow; PCV, preset inspiratory pressure, backup rate, I:E ratio or inspiratory time
- For PSV: preset inspiratory pressure
- Adjust F_{IO_2} and PEEP; usual goal $Pa_{O_2} > 55$ mm Hg, O_2 saturation $>90\%$; adjust minute ventilation to achieve Pa_{CO_2} needed for pH between 7.32 and 7.45 (unless contraindications)

■ Pearl

Using a low tidal volume (6–8 mL/kg ideal weight) improves outcome in ARDS, asthma, and COPD patients, possibly because of decreased lung injury and barotrauma.

Reference

Tobin MJ: Advances in mechanical ventilation. N Engl J Med 2001;344:1986. [PMID: 11430329]

Mechanical Ventilation in ARDS

- **Essential Concepts**
  - Lung injury diffuse but nonhomogeneous, ranging from completely normal areas to severely atelectatic regions
  - Oxygenation goal: Increase FIO_2 and PEEP as needed to achieve $PaO_2 > 55$ mm Hg, but minimize O_2 toxicity by keeping $FIO_2 < 0.4$ and using PEEP judiciously to avoid complications
  - PEEP increases end-expiratory lung volume, keeping lung units from collapsing and may "recruit" collapsed lung units
  - Mechanical ventilation counters high work of breathing with low compliance lungs
  - Low tidal volume ($VT = 6$ mL/kg ideal weight) strategy minimizes lung damage; improves survival, lessens barotrauma and cardiovascular compromise, but may result in hypercapnia

- **Essentials of Management**
  - Volume-cycled ventilation preferred; alternative pressure-controlled ventilation
  - Tidal volume (VT) at 6 mL/kg ideal weight; keep inspiratory plateau pressure < 30 cm H_2O, if necessary, lower V_T to 4–5 mL/kg
  - Respiratory rate up to 35/min with goal pH 7.30–7.45; if pH < 7.30 and rate $= 35$, consider sodium bicarbonate; if pH < 7.15, consider increased VT
  - Use least of these FIO_2/PEEP combinations to achieve PaO_2 55–80 mm Hg: FIO_2 0.4/PEEP 5 cm H_2O, 0.4/8, 0.5/8, 0.5/10, 0.6/10, 0.7/10, 0.7/12, 0.7/14, 0.8/14, 0.9/16, 0.9/18, 1.0/18–25
  - Check daily chest radiographs for endotracheal tube position, evidence of barotrauma

- **Pearl**

A low tidal volume strategy (VT 6 mL/kg or less) is the only therapy shown to improve outcome in ARDS.

Reference

The Acute Respiratory Distress Syndrome Network. Ventilation with lower tidal volumes as compared with traditional tidal volumes for acute lung injury and the acute respiratory distress syndrome. N Engl J Med 2000; 342:1301. [PMID: 10793162]

Mechanical Ventilation in Neuromuscular Disorders

- ■ Essential Concepts
  - • Hypercapnia often seen with vital capacity < 55% predicted or < 15 mL/kg
  - • Generally requires mechanical ventilation when hypercapnia develops, especially if disease progressive or worsening
  - • Patients with respiratory muscle weakness prone to impaired cough, poor mucociliary clearance of secretions, pneumonia
  - • Hypoxemia due to atelectasis, mucous plugging of airways, pneumonia; usually absence of increased airway resistance and abnormal lung mechanics

- ■ Essentials of Management
  - • Consider mechanical ventilation in patient with progressive neuromuscular weakness with V_T < 15 mL/kg and falling; $PaCO_2$ > 50 mm Hg and rising; unresponsive to other treatments; central nervous system disorder with central hypoventilation unresponsive to treatment
  - • Volume-cycled ventilation
  - • Tidal volume (V_T) 6–8 mL/kg ideal weight to start, keep inspiratory plateau pressure < 30 cm H_2O.
  - • Adjust respiratory rate to maintain pH 7.35–7.45
  - • PEEP to help prevent or reverse atelectasis from breathing at low lung volumes
  - • Frequent suctioning, postural drainage, chest percussion (if indicated)
  - • Patients with ventilatory control disorders (central hypoventilation) may not "trigger" ventilator adequately
  - • Daily chest radiographs for endotracheal tube position, evidence of barotrauma
  - • Consider noninvasive positive pressure ventilation (NIPPV), if acute reversible neurological disorder, mild respiratory failure, patient awake, alert

- ■ Pearl

Ventilator-associated pneumonia frequently complicates respiratory failure from neuromuscular diseases.

Reference

MacDuff A, Grant IS: Critical care management of neuromuscular disease, including long-term ventilation. Curr Opin Crit Care 2003;9:106. [PMID: 12657972]

Mechanical Ventilation in Status Asthmaticus

- **Essential Concepts**
  - Mechanical ventilation may be needed because of respiratory muscle fatigue, especially because reversal of airway obstruction may take hours to days
  - Patients with severe hyperinflation have very high end-inspiratory and high end-expiratory volume; therefore at risk for barotrauma, hypotension, respiratory acidosis
  - Goal to minimize hyperinflation by maximizing expiratory time (low respiratory rate), minimizing inspiratory time (low tidal volume, high inspiratory flow rates)
  - Reduction of hyperinflation improves gas exchange and decreases work of breathing
  - May accept mild-to-moderate hypercapnia to meet goals

- **Essentials of Management**
  - Indications: Status asthmaticus with severe acidosis; very high work of breathing, heavy airway secretions, impending inspiratory muscle failure
  - Maximize pharmacotherapy: bronchodilators, corticosteroids
  - Volume-cycled ventilation; set tidal volume (V_T) 6–8 mL/kg ideal weight; use inspiratory flow rate 70–100 L/min to minimize inspiratory time
  - Goals: inspiratory plateau pressure <25–30 cm H_2O, I:E ratio at least 1:3 (preferably 1:4–5), low intrinsic PEEP (<5 cm H_2O)
  - Low V_T and respiratory rate combination may lead to hypercapnia; hypercapnia acceptable if pH > 7.25
  - Daily chest radiographs for endotracheal tube position, evidence of barotrauma

- **Pearl**

As long as hyperinflation is avoided, be patient with status asthmaticus and mechanical ventilation; it may take 3–7 days or even more for airway inflammation to resolve.

Reference

Peigang Y et al: Ventilation of patients with asthma and chronic obstructive pulmonary disease. Curr Opin Crit Care 2002;8:70. [PMID: 12205409]

Mechanical Ventilation, Complications of

- ■ Essentials of Diagnosis
  - • Pulmonary: barotrauma, such as pneumothorax, pneumomediastinum, acute lung injury, hypo- or hyperventilation, ventilator-associated pneumonia, atelectasis, rarely O_2 toxicity
  - • Extrapulmonary: hemodynamic, such as hypotension, low cardiac output, impaired venous return; increased intracranial pressure (mild), psychological dependence on ventilator; multiorgan system failure; misinterpretation of intravascular pressures measured inside thorax (pulmonary artery or central venous catheter)

- ■ Differential Diagnosis
  - • Nosocomial infection, including pneumonia
  - • Sepsis
  - • Hypovolemia
  - • Cardiac tamponade
  - • Pulmonary thromboembolism
  - • Cardiogenic pulmonary edema, noncardiogenic pulmonary edema, transfusion-associated lung injury
  - • Pneumothorax or pneumomediastinum from catheter placement, ruptured esophagus

- ■ Treatment
  - • Anticipate complications with daily chest radiograph (pneumothorax), follow arterial blood gases
  - • Suspect positive-pressure ventilation if hypotension, low cardiac output (oliguria, prerenal azotemia, hypotension), pneumothorax, pneumomediastinum
  - • If hypotension or low cardiac output, consider volume challenge, 250–500 mL of 0.9% NaCl, monitor CVP and blood pressure
  - • Use low tidal volume (VT 6–8 mL/kg) combined with adequate respiratory rate to achieve goal $Paco_2$ and Pao_2 to minimize barotrauma risk
  - • Suspect ventilator-associated pneumonia if fever, infiltrates on chest radiograph, >3 days of mechanical ventilation

- ■ Pearl

Oxygen toxicity is associated with prolonged use of 100% O_2, but is considered unlikely with $F_{IO_2} < 0.50$.

Reference

Tobin MJ: Advances in mechanical ventilation. N Engl J Med 2001;344:1986.
    [PMID: 11430329]

Mechanical Ventilation, Failure to Wean from

- **Essentials of Diagnosis**
  - Excessive dyspnea or hypercapnia, hypoxemia when ventilatory support withdrawn; often imbalance between ventilatory requirement and inadequate capacity
  - Anticipate if minute ventilation ($\dot{V}E$) on ventilator >12 L/min, spontaneous rate/VT (L) >100, spontaneous $\dot{V}E$ < 6 L/min, vital capacity <15 mL/kg

- **Differential Diagnosis**
  - High $\dot{V}E$ requirement (>12 L/min): fever, metabolic acidosis, renal failure, agitation, activity, infection, hyperthyroidism, administration of excessive calories (especially carbohydrate), lung or heart disease (high dead space/tidal volume ratio).
  - Low $\dot{V}E$ capacity (spontaneous $\dot{V}E$ < 6 L/min): neuromuscular weakness (critical illness polyneuropathy or myopathy), malnutrition, hypophosphatemia, hypokalemia, primary muscle disease, diaphragmatic weakness, flail chest, rib fractures, ascites, abdominal distension, pain, high resistance of endotracheal tube (<7.0 mm)

- **Treatment**
  - Wean when $\dot{V}E$ < 10–12 L/min; patient afebrile, stable hemodynamically; normal serum potassium and phosphorus, adequate nutritional support, minimal respiratory secretions, little or no bronchospasm, no pulmonary edema, serum bicarbonate >18 mmol/L
  - Relieve severe ascites or abdominal distension, abdominal or chest wall pain (especially if with respiration)
  - If stable, perform daily spontaneous breathing trial; respiratory rate/tidal volume (L) <60, predicts successful weaning; >110 predicts failure; 60–110, marginal predictive value
  - Correct electrolytes; consider malnutrition, neuropathy or myopathy, diaphragmatic fatigue or paralysis; avoid excessive sedation
  - Transient noninvasive positive pressure ventilation helpful after extubation

- **Pearl**

Routine daily trials of spontaneous breathing in stable patients decreases length of stay in ICU and duration of mechanical ventilation.

Reference

MacIntyre NR et al: Evidence-based guidelines for weaning and discontinuing ventilatory support. Chest 2001;120(6 Suppl):375S. [PMID: 11742959]

Noninvasive Positive Pressure Ventilation (NIPPV)

■ Essential Concepts

- Delivery of positive-pressure ventilation without endotracheal tube via nasal or oronasal facemask; success depends on alert, cooperative patient with proper fitting interface
- Continuous positive airway pressure (CPAP): delivers constant pressure during both inspiration and expiration
- Bilevel devices: cycle between two different positive pressures; inspiratory pressure (IPAP) set higher than expiratory pressure (EPAP)
- Useful in select patients with acute or chronic respiratory failure
- Obstructive sleep apnea (OSA): maintains upper airway patency
- COPD: improves gas exchange, vital signs, dyspnea scores; reduces need for invasive mechanical ventilation
- Weaning from invasive mechanical ventilation: shorter duration of support, fewer ICU days, improved 60-day mortality
- Pulmonary edema: afterload reduction and improved cardiac output achieved by lowering left ventricular transmural pressure
- Contraindications: acute respiratory arrest, ischemia, hypotensive shock, uncontrolled arrhythmias, excessive secretions, inability to protect airway, facial abnormalities
- Complications: nasal bridge skin breakdown, sinus congestion, sinusitis, dry eyes, dry mouth, headache, gastric distention

■ Essentials of Management

- OSA: CPAP treatment of choice; if unable to tolerate high pressure levels required to maintain airway patency switch to bilevel device adjusting EPAP level until obstructive apneas abolished; adjust IPAP level to reduce hypopneas, desaturations, snoring
- COPD: Bilevel devices with high IPAP to reduce work of inspiratory muscles and EPAP lower than intrinsic PEEP
- Pulmonary edema: CPAP starting at 10–12.5 cm H_2O; caution with bilevel modes until further studies available

■ Pearl

Patients are not subject to the potential complications of intubation, loss of airway defense mechanisms, and self-extubation with the use of NIPPV compared to invasive mechanical ventilation.

Reference

Liesching T et al: Acute applications of noninvasive positive pressure ventilation. Chest 2003 Aug;124:699. [PMID: 1290756]

Positive End-Expiratory Pressure (PEEP)

■ Essential Concepts

- PEEP given with positive-pressure ventilation or as continuous positive airway pressure (CPAP)
- Normally, exhalation continues until alveolar equals atmospheric pressure (0 cm H_2O); end-expiratory lung volume determined by lung and chest wall compliance
- If PEEP applied, end-expiratory alveolar pressure then equals PEEP; thereby increasing end-expiratory volume, which decreases or reverses atelectasis, adding lung participating in gas exchange
- PEEP decreases RV and LV preload, increases RV but decreases LV afterload; may reduce cardiac output; contributes to hypotension, organ hypoperfusion
- Cardiovascular effects most if lungs normal or more compliant; smaller effects with stiff lungs

■ Essentials of Management

- Use PEEP for hypoxemia in ARDS, pulmonary edema, atelectasis; may be helpful for patients with low lung volume (obesity, postsurgery, neuromuscular weakness, ascites)
- Usually avoid with hypotension, volume depletion, increased intracranial pressure, obstructive lung disease
- Use least PEEP to improve hypoxemia, minimize inspired O_2 concentration, reduce or reverse atelectasis
- One protocol for FIO_2 and PEEP in ARDS—use least FIO_2/PEEP combination to achieve PaO_2 55–80 mm Hg: FIO_2 0.4/PEEP 5 cm H_2O, 0.4/8, 0.5/8, 0.5/10, 0.6/10, 0.7/10, 0.7/12, 0.7/14, 0.8/14, 0.9/16, 0.9/18, 1.0/18–25
- For other disorders, optimal PEEP not known, but can use same for ARDS
- Consider lower levels of PEEP for nonhomogeneous atelectasis, hypotension, low cardiac output
- Adverse effects of PEEP: hypotension, low cardiac output, decreased nonrespiratory organ failure, pneumothorax, pneumomediastinum

■ Pearl

Both high PEEP and low tidal volume or low PEEP and high tidal volume can damage the lungs.

Reference

Gattinoni L et al: Physiologic rationale for ventilator setting in acute lung injury/acute respiratory distress syndrome patients. Crit Care Med 2003;31(4 Suppl):S300. [PMID: 12682456]

Respiratory Failure from Chronic Obstructive Lung Disease

- **Essentials of Diagnosis**
  - Chronic bronchitis or emphysema
  - Increasing dyspnea, often with cough, decreased exercise capacity, increased sputum production, respiratory muscle fatigue
  - Mild to moderate hypoxemia; may have $PaCO_2$ >50 mm Hg with acute respiratory acidosis (pH < 7.35), even in those without chronic CO_2 retention
  - Mechanisms include increased airway resistance (bronchospasm, increased secretions, airway edema), infection and host response to infection (change in bacterial type, purulent sputum), altered lung mechanics (hyperinflation)

- **Differential Diagnosis**
  - Asthma, pneumonia, pulmonary edema
  - Neuromuscular weakness or central hypoventilation syndrome

- **Treatment**
  - Identify most severe: very low peak expiratory flow, pH < 7.25 with $PaCO_2$ >60, right heart failure, pneumothorax, pneumonia, poor response to bronchodilators, malnutrition, multiorgan failure
  - Oxygen: 2–4 L/min nasal cannula or FIO_2 0.28–0.40 by Venturi mask
  - Aerosolized albuterol and ipratropium bromide; theophylline not recommended
  - Intravenous or oral corticosteroids; taper 7–10 days
  - Antibiotics against *S pneumoniae, H influenzae, M catarrhalis* (2nd generation cephalosporins, extended-spectrum macrolides, fluoroquinolones)
  - In selected patients, noninvasive positive pressure ventilation up to 12–24 hours
  - Mechanical ventilation if severe, nonresponse to therapy, altered mental status, muscle fatigue

- **Pearl**

Patients with most severe hypoxemia and lowest pH (acute respiratory acidosis) are at highest risk for worsening hypercapnia with administration of oxygen.

Reference

Bach PB et al: Management of acute exacerbations of chronic obstructive pulmonary disease: a summary and appraisal of published evidence. Ann Intern Med 2001;134:600. [PMID: 11281745]

Respiratory Failure from Neuromuscular Disorders

- **Essentials of Diagnosis**
  - Weakness of respiratory muscles or dysfunction of ventilatory control from neuromuscular or neurological disease
  - $Paco_2 > 50$ mm Hg, usually with additional hypoxemia
  - If weakness, vital capacity (VC) <1500 mL associated with hypercapnia
  - Disorders of ventilatory control due to sedative or opioid overdose, head trauma, brain stem stroke, hypothyroidism, poliomyelitis
  - Respiratory muscle weakness due to spinal cord disease (trauma, cancer, paraspinous abscess, amyotrophic lateral sclerosis); neuropathic disease (myasthenia gravis, botulism, Guillain-Barré syndrome, tick paralysis, drugs, peripheral neuropathy); primary muscle disease (polymyositis, endocrinopathies, hypophosphatemia, hypokalemia); ICU patients (critical illness polyneuropathy or polymyopathy); extremity strength may not reflect strength of respiratory muscles

- **Differential Diagnosis**
  - Primary lung disease with acquired neuromuscular weakness (critical illness polyneuropathy)
  - Chest wall deformity or abnormality

- **Treatment**
  - Treat underlying disease
  - Oxygen for hypoxemia due to atelectasis or pneumonia
  - Consider endotracheal intubation and mechanical ventilation when VC<15 mL/kg or 1200 mL in adults, especially if worsening
  - Patients with weakness have disproportionate atelectasis, inability to clear secretions and pneumonia, pulmonary thromboembolic disease

- **Pearl**

Suspect acquired neuromuscular weakness due to critical illness polyneuropathy or myopathy in a patient who fails to wean from mechanical ventilation.

Reference

Rabinstein AA et al: Warning signs of imminent respiratory failure in neurological patients. Semin Neurol 2003;23:97. [PMID: 12870111]

Respiratory Failure from Thoracic Cage Disorders

- Essentials of Diagnosis
  - Structural or functional abnormality of chest wall or diaphragm
  - $Paco_2 > 50$ mm Hg, usually with hypoxemia
  - Some disorders limit chest expansion (restriction), such as kyphoscoliosis or ankylosing spondylitis, pleural effusions, restrictive pleuritis
  - Truncal obesity, pregnancy, ascites, severe abdominal organomegaly, recent abdominal surgery limit diaphragmatic excursion
  - Severe chronic thoracic cage disorders may lead to pulmonary hypertension and cor pulmonale
  - Severely obese patients have a high likelihood of obstructive sleep apnea (OSA) and obesity hypoventilation syndrome (OHS)

- Differential Diagnosis
  - Primary lung diseases (COPD, asthma, interstitial lung disease)
  - Neuromuscular disease with respiratory muscle weakness

- Treatment
  - Treat underlying disease
  - Oxygen for hypoxemia due to atelectasis or pneumonia
  - Endotracheal intubation and mechanical ventilation for hypercapnia; may try noninvasive positive pressure ventilation if mild, reversible cause

- Pearl

Patients with weakness have disproportionate atelectasis, inability to clear secretions and pneumonia (frequent suctioning and mobilization of secretions), and pulmonary thromboembolic disease compared to other chest wall disorders.

Reference

Goldstein RS: Hypoventilation: neuromuscular and chest wall disorders. Clin Chest Med 1992;13:507. [PMID: 1521416]

Respiratory Failure: Arterial Hypercapnia

- **Essentials of Diagnosis**
  - Arterial $Paco_2$ ($Paco_2$) >45 mm Hg, with pH < 7.35
  - May have headache, bradycardia, confusion, lethargy, or coma
  - Other features depend on presence of hypoxemia or features of underlying disease
  - May be seen with severe pulmonary diseases
  - Nonpulmonary causes of respiratory failure often have hypercapnia, such as disorders of ventilatory control or chest wall, neuromuscular diseases

- **Differential Diagnosis**
  - Severe COPD, status asthmaticus, interstitial lung diseases, pulmonary edema
  - Head injury, stroke, brain stem dysfunction, sedative overdose impairing ventilatory control
  - Neuromuscular disorders affecting respiratory muscles, such as phrenic nerve injury, brain stem stroke, myasthenia gravis, Guillain-Barré syndrome, metabolic muscle diseases, electrolyte disorders, critical illness polyneuropathy or polymyopathy
  - Chest wall or diaphragmatic weakness, injury, or diseases

- **Treatment**
  - Establish patent airway (positioning, suctioning, artificial airway)
  - Measure Pao_2 to assess oxygenation status
  - Treat underlying disease
  - Provide adequate ventilation to achieve goal $Paco_2$ for pH >7.35 (unless contraindicated)
  - Endotracheal intubation, mechanical ventilation if necessary; in selected patients, noninvasive positive pressure ventilation useful

- **Pearl**

Use formula to determine minute ventilation ($\dot{V}E$) needed: $\dot{V}E = 863 \times VCO_2/[Paco_2 \times (1 - VD/VT)]$ where $\dot{V}E$ is minute ventilation (L/min); $\dot{V}CO_2$ is CO_2 output (L/min); VD/VT is dead-space/tidal volume ratio.

Reference

Epstein SK et al: Respiratory acidosis. Respir Care 2001;46:366. [PMID: 11262556]

Respiratory Failure: Hypoxemia

- Essentials of Diagnosis
  - Arterial P_{O_2} (Pa_{O_2}) <60 mm Hg, equivalent to arterial O_2 saturation <92%
  - If Pa_{O_2} is less than expected when breathing supplemental O_2 (F_{IO_2} >21%), should also consider as hypoxemia
  - May have tachycardia, tachypnea, diaphoresis, anxiety, cyanosis, arrhythmias
  - If severe, may have confusion, lethargy, or coma
  - May coexist with respiratory acidosis (Pa_{CO_2} >45 mm Hg with pH < 7.35); may have respiratory depression, impaired level of consciousness
  - Any pulmonary disease, pneumonia, COPD, asthma, pulmonary embolism, ARDS, atelectasis, interstitial lung diseases; also pleural effusions, pulmonary edema, extrapulmonary right-to-left shunt

- Differential Diagnosis
  - Decreased O_2 delivery—low cardiac output, shock, anemia—without arterial hypoxemia (i.e. normal Pa_{O_2})
  - Carboxyhemoglobinemia

- Treatment
  - Establish airway (positioning, suctioning, artificial airway)
  - Measure Pa_{CO_2} to assess ventilation status
  - Supplemental O_2; amount based on likely disease and mechanism of hypoxemia; goal Pa_{O_2} >60 mm Hg or O_2 saturation >92%
  - Asthma, COPD, pulmonary embolism, mild pneumonia and atelectasis respond to F_{IO_2} 0.24–0.4 (usually caused by $\dot{V}/\dot{Q}$ mismatching)
  - ARDS, severe pneumonia or atelectasis, and extracardiac right-to-left shunts require F_{IO_2} 0.4–1.0 (due to hypoxemia from right-to-left shunts)
  - Endotracheal intubation, PEEP and mechanical ventilation needed if severe

- Pearl

You cannot predict the new Pa_{O_2} when you change the F_{IO_2} because Pa_{O_2} depends on the mechanism of hypoxemia.

Reference

Henig NR et al: Mechanisms of hypoxemia. Respir Care Clin N Am 2000;6:501. [PMID: 11172576]

Status Asthmaticus

- **Essentials of Diagnosis**
  - Severe asthma (severely reduced peak flow, FEV_1, VC) poorly or nonresponsive to therapy
  - Hypoxemia; may have hypercapnia with acute respiratory acidosis
  - Poor air movement, severe wheezing but wheezing absent when very severe, hyperinflation, use of accessory muscles of respiration, pulsus paradoxus
  - Associated with worsening asthma and increasing bronchodilator use over days, but may develop suddenly without warning

- **Differential Diagnosis**
  - Acute upper airway obstruction (larnygeal edema, angioedema, tumor, foreign body, trauma, epiglottis)
  - Vocal cord dysfunction syndrome
  - COPD exacerbation
  - Cardiogenic pulmonary edema, pneumothorax, pulmonary embolism, pneumonia

- **Treatment**
  - Oxygen, 2–4 L/min nasal cannula or 40–60% by mask, to achieve PaO_2 >60–70 mm Hg
  - Inhaled bronchodilators: albuterol every 20–30 minutes; then hourly; ipratropium bromide every 2–4 hours
  - Systemic corticosteroids: prednisone, 40–60 mg, 1–4 times per day; or IV methylprednisolone, 20–40 mg every 6 hours
  - If needed, noninvasive positive pressure ventilation; endotracheal intubation and mechanical ventilation
  - Antibiotics not usually indicated; but consider if purulent sputum, fever, pneumonia
  - Other therapy: IV magnesium sulfate (2–8 g IV every 4 hours) may benefit very severe asthma; no clear role for leukotriene modifiers, inhaled corticosteroids

- **Pearl**

Because airway inflammation, not bronchospasm, is the cause of status asthmaticus, be patient; several days might be needed before obstruction reverses.

Reference

McFadden ER Jr: Acute severe asthma. Am J Respir Crit Care Med 2003;168:740 [PMID: 14522812]

Ventilator-Associated Pneumonia

- **Essentials of Diagnosis**
  - In patient on mechanical ventilation, three or more of fever, new infiltrates, leukocytosis, purulent secretions
  - Occurs in 10–25% of mechanically ventilated patients, resulting in 5–30% increase in mortality; increased duration of ventilation
  - Due to aspiration of bacterial-laden oropharyngeal secretions or gastric contents through or around endotracheal tube and cuff
  - Community-acquired bacteria if pneumonia occurs <4 days after admission; otherwise Gram-negative bacilli, staphylococcus more common
  - Culture of sputum helpful for antibiotic selection, not for diagnosis; contamination-protected brushes, bronchoscopic sampling, or bronchoalveolar lavage possibly helpful if quantitative cultures used

- **Differential Diagnosis**
  - Community-acquired pneumonia
  - Pulmonary edema, ARDS
  - Aspiration pneumonitis
  - Atelectasis
  - Pulmonary thromboembolism

- **Treatment**
  - Suction secretions, chest physical therapy (only if increase in sputum production)
  - Antibiotics directed against community-acquired organisms (*S pneumoniae, H influenzae*) if <4 days; if >4 days, antibiotics against aerobic Gram-negative bacilli, (*E coli, K pneumoniae, Pseudomonas, Acinetobacter*) and *S aureus*
  - Plan to reduce spectrum of antibiotic coverage within 3–7 days using clinical response, cultures, epidemiology of bacteria in ICU
  - Prevention: Suction secretions above endotracheal tube cuff; continuous enteral feedings

- **Pearl**

Noninvasive positive pressure ventilation is associated with decreased risk of infection.

Reference

Hoffken G et al: Nosocomial pneumonia: the importance of a deescalating strategy for antibiotic treatment of pneumonia in the ICU. Chest 2002;122:2183. [PMID: 12475862]

Cardiology

Angina Pectoris

- **Essentials of Diagnosis**
  - Heavy, pressure-like substernal chest discomfort; precipitated by exertion or stress; lasting <15 minutes; relieved with rest or nitroglycerin
  - Radiation to left arm, neck, or jaw; dyspnea, nausea
  - Examination usually benign; may detect gallop or mitral regurgitation murmur during anginal event
  - ECG varies between normal and ST segment depression; increased specificity when dynamic ST segment changes occur with symptoms
  - Different stress testing modalities available for diagnostic purpose
  - Coronary angiography provides anatomical roadmap to guide therapy

- **Differential Diagnosis**
  - Cardiovascular: unstable angina, myocardial infarction, Prinzmetal angina, pericarditis, myocarditis, aortic dissection
  - Pulmonary: pneumothorax, pulmonary embolism, pneumonia
  - Gastrointestinal: esophageal reflux or spasm, gastritis, peptic ulcer disease, cholangitis, hepatitis, pancreatitis
  - Musculoskeletal pain and costochondritis

- **Treatment**
  - Increase oxygen supply and reduce myocardial oxygen demand
  - Rapid administration of aspirin
  - Reduce heart rate and blood pressure with beta-blockers
  - Nitrates for symptom relief
  - Oxygen
  - Calcium channel blockers are negative inotropes and coronary vasodilators; may be used for patients unable to tolerate beta-blockade
  - Angioplasty with possible stenting indicated for persistent symptoms on optimal medical management
  - Long-term recommendations for behavioral modification, blood pressure control, addition of HMG-CoA reductase inhibitors

- **Pearl**

Except for left main or three-vessel disease with left ventricular dysfunction, angioplasty and coronary artery bypass graft surgery (CABG) have not yet demonstrated benefits in mortality reduction.

Reference

Gibbons RJ et al: ACC/AHA 2002 guideline update for the management of patients with chronic stable angina. Circulation 2003;107:149. [PMID: 12515758]

Aortic Dissection, Acute

- **Essentials of Diagnosis**
  - Abrupt onset of severe, tearing chest pain radiating to back; reaches maximal intensity immediately
  - Symptoms related to area of arterial compromise: paraplegia (anterior spinal), stroke (carotid), abdominal pain (mesenteric), tamponade (proximal aorta)
  - Dizziness, dyspnea, oliguria
  - Tachycardia, unequal blood pressures in upper extremities, murmur of aortic insufficiency
  - Myocardial infarction from coronary ostia involvement rare
  - Chest radiograph with widened mediastinum
  - CT and MRI highly sensitive and specific; transesophageal echocardiogram if imaging not feasible
  - Aortography carries significant risk and time delay
  - Risk factors: hypertension, Marfan/Ehlers-Danlos syndromes, coarctation, bicuspid aortic valve, aortitis (syphilis), age 60–80, pregnancy, cardiac catheterization, intra-aortic balloon pump, trauma

- **Differential Diagnosis**
  - Acute myocardial infarction
  - Angina pectoris
  - Pneumothorax
  - Acute pericarditis
  - Boerhaave syndrome
  - Pulmonary embolism

- **Treatment**
  - Close hemodynamic monitoring with goal to decrease systolic blood pressure and sheer forces across aortic wall
  - Labetalol drug of choice to reduce sheer forces
  - Calcium-channel blockers alternative for beta-blockers
  - Vasodilators (nitroprusside, nitroglycerin, hydralazine) for blood pressure control once adequate beta-blockade achieved
  - Pain control
  - Avoid anticoagulation and thrombolytics
  - Surgical repair for Stanford Type A dissection (involves ascending aortic arch); Stanford Type B (distal to take-off of last great vessel) managed medically unless rupture, limb or organ ischemia, persistent pain, saccular aneurysm formation

- **Pearl**

The mortality rate from untreated acute aortic dissection is estimated to be approximately 1% per hour.

Reference

Erbel R et al: Diagnosis and management of aortic dissection. Eur Heart J 2001;22:1642. [PMID: 11511117]

Aortic Valvular Heart Disease

- **Essentials of Diagnosis**
  - Dyspnea, orthopnea, paroxysmal nocturnal dyspnea, cough, syncope, chest pain; signs and symptoms differ between acute and chronic lesions
  - Aortic stenosis (AS): angina, syncope, pulsus parvus et tardus, harsh crescendo-decrescendo systolic murmur; may be due to rheumatic heart disease, congenital abnormalities, calcification
  - Aortic regurgitation (AR): wide pulse pressure, water-hammer pulse, Quincke pulse, Duroziez sign, early diastolic murmur; may be due to leaflet disorders (endocarditis, myxomatous degeneration, bicuspid valve) or dilated aortic root (syphilis, aortic dissection, connective tissue disorders)
  - Echocardiogram essential in confirming and assessing diagnosis

- **Differential Diagnosis**
  - Aortic stenosis: mitral regurgitation, hypertrophic cardiomyopathy (HCM), ventricular septal defect (VSD)
  - Aortic regurgitation: mitral stenosis, pulmonary hypertension with Graham-Steele murmur

- **Treatment**
  - Aortic stenosis: no medical management; when severe, requires surgery or valvuloplasty (transiently effective); vasodilator drugs may cause severe hypotension
  - Aortic regurgitation: diuretics with sodium and fluid restriction; digoxin; preload and afterload reduction with ACE inhibitors, hydralazine plus nitrates, nitroprusside
  - Infective endocarditis prophylaxis
  - Cardiac catheterization often necessary prior to surgery
  - Surgical valve repair or replacement ideally indicated for all symptomatic patients

- **Pearl**

Symptomatic aortic stenosis confers a poor prognosis with the average time to death often limited to only a few years: with angina—3 years, syncope—3 years, and pulmonary edema—2 years.

Reference

Bonow RO et al: ACC/AHA guidelines for the management of patients with valvular heart disease. J Am Coll Cardiol 1998;32:1486. [PMID: 9809971]

Arterial Insufficiency, Acute

- **Essentials of Diagnosis**
  - Sudden reduction or cessation of blood flow to peripheral artery followed by ischemic insult with severe localized pain
  - Affected limb pale, cool, mottled; distal pulse absent
  - Numbness common; paralysis late sign
  - Compartment syndrome from excessive muscle necrosis and swelling
  - Doppler exam and ankle-brachial index (ABI) helpful screening tools
  - Arteriography remains standard for diagnosis and locates extent of occlusion
  - Usually caused by arterial emboli (from heart) or thrombosis; often in setting of atrial fibrillation

- **Differential Diagnosis**
  - Deep venous thrombosis with phlegmasia alba dolens
  - Heparin-induced thrombocytopenia syndrome (HITS)
  - Hypoperfusion and shock states
  - Atheroembolism: cholesterol emboli
  - Peripheral neuropathic pain
  - Aortic dissection or aneurysm
  - Vasculitis

- **Treatment**
  - Goal to restore blood supply to compromised area
  - Immediate anticoagulation with heparin; unless HITS suspected
  - Surgical thromboembolectomy treatment of choice
  - Fasciotomy if compartment syndrome develops
  - Intra-arterial thrombolytics for acute thrombosis especially in nonoperable lesions
  - Correct electrolyte and acid-base disturbances especially postreperfusion
  - Monitor for rhabdomyolysis and renal failure
  - Mannitol to reduce cellular edema and prevent myoglobin induced renal failure
  - Pain control

- **Pearl**

The "six-Ps" commonly associated with acute arterial insufficiency are pain, paralysis, paresthesias, pallor, pulselessness, and poikilothermia.

Reference

Henke PK et al: Approach to the patient with acute limb ischemia: diagnosis and therapeutic modalities. Cardiol Clin 2002;20:513. [PMID: 12472039]

Atrial Fibrillation

■ Essentials of Diagnosis

- Irregularly occurring irregular heart beat with loss of synchronized atrial rhythm and irregular ventricular response
- Chest pain, dyspnea, palpitations, dizziness
- Acute onset may lead to hypotension, myocardial ischemia, acute congestive heart failure, hypoperfusion to end-organs
- Embolic symptoms may be seen in chronic atrial fibrillation: stroke, ischemic limb, mesenteric ischemia, renal impairment
- ECG with fibrillatory waves, loss of P waves, irregular QRS intervals, rapid ventricular rate
- Etiologies: alcohol, hyperthyroidism, mitral valve disease, ischemic heart disease, hypokalemia, hypomagnesemia, sepsis, pericarditis, post–cardiac surgery, idiopathic

■ Differential Diagnosis

- Atrial flutter with variable block
- Multifocal atrial tachycardia
- Atrial tachycardia with variable block
- Atrioventricular nodal reentrant tachycardia
- Sinus arrhythmia
- Pre-excitation/accessory pathway
- Normal sinus rhythm with multiple premature atrial contractions

■ Treatment

- Identify underlying etiology and precipitating factors
- Immediate electrical countershock if hemodynamic compromise
- Rate control with digoxin, beta-blockers, Ca-channel blockers; avoid excessive AV nodal blockade
- Anticoagulation if not contraindicated
- May cardiovert without anticoagulation if onset <48 hours; otherwise, anticoagulate and cardiovert in 4 weeks
- Can cardiovert sooner if transesophageal echocardiogram without thrombus; continue anticoagulation for 4 weeks
- Cardioversion may be electrical or pharmacologic (type Ia, Ic, III antiarrhythmics)
- Echocardiogram to evaluate valvular lesions, chamber sizes, thrombus formation

■ Pearl

The "atrial kick" contributes to about 20% of the cardiac output. The loss of the atrial kick, as in atrial fibrillation, can be significant in patients with already reduced systolic function.

Reference

Fuster V et al: ACC/AHA/ESC guidelines for the management of patients with atrial fibrillation. Circulation 2001;104:2118. [PMID: 11673357]

Cardiac Tamponade

- **Essentials of Diagnosis**
  - Beck triad: hypotension, elevated jugular venous pressure (JVP), muffled heart sounds
  - Pleuritic chest pain, dyspnea, orthopnea, palpitations, oliguria
  - Tachycardia, pericardial rub, pulsus paradoxus, peripheral edema, distended neck veins
  - Kussmaul sign: increased JVP with inspiration; nonspecific
  - Chest radiograph may not show enlarged cardiac silhouette (water-bottle shaped heart) if acute onset
  - ECG with reduced voltages, electrical alternans
  - Echocardiogram with pericardial effusion, "swinging heart," right atrial systolic or ventricular diastolic collapse
  - Pulmonary artery catheterization with equalization of pressures: right atrial, left atrial, left ventricular end-diastolic
  - Pericardial effusion compromises ventricular filling with reduced cardiac output
  - Etiologies: uremia, pericarditis, malignancy, infection (viral, bacterial, fungal, tuberculosis), myocardial infarction/rupture, trauma, idiopathic, hypothyroidism, anticoagulation (especially post–cardiac surgery)

- **Differential Diagnosis**
  - Constrictive pericarditis
  - Tension pneumothorax
  - Right ventricular infarction
  - Restrictive cardiomyopathy
  - End-stage cardiac failure

- **Treatment**
  - Volume resuscitation for hypotension; dopamine if blood pressure does not improve with fluids
  - Pericardiocentesis with or without pigtail catheter drainage
  - Hemodynamic monitoring with pulmonary artery catheter
  - Treat underlying cause of pericardial effusion
  - Surgical pericardial window (pericardiectomy or balloon pericardiotomy) if recurrent accumulation
  - Positive pressure ventilation may worsen symptoms

- **Pearl**

The "rule of 20s" in cardiac tamponade: CVP >20 mm Hg, HR increase >20 beats per minute, pulsus paradoxus >20, systolic BP, decrease >20 mm Hg, and pulse pressure <20.

Reference

Spodick DH: Acute cardiac tamponade. N Engl J Med 2003;349:684. [PMID: 12917306]

Congestive Heart Failure

- **Essentials of Diagnosis**
  - Shortness of breath, dyspnea on exertion, orthopnea, paroxysmal nocturnal dyspnea, weight gain, leg swelling, pink frothy sputum
  - Tachypnea, inspiratory crepitations, gallops, cyanosis, peripheral edema
  - Chest radiograph with pulmonary edema, pleural effusions, cardiomegaly
  - Elevated B-type natriuretic peptide, hypoxemia, metabolic acidosis
  - Echocardiogram or right heart catheterization with reduced ejection fraction (systolic dysfunction) or inadequate diastolic filling (diastolic dysfunction)

- **Differential Diagnosis**
  - Noncardiogenic pulmonary edema: ARDS
  - Valvular heart disease • Pericardial disease
  - Hypoalbumin states • Fluid overload
  - Hypothyroidism and myxedema
  - Pulmonary vascular disease

- **Treatment**
  - Acute left ventricular failure: oxygen; preload and afterload reduction: nitrates, nitroprusside, morphine; diuresis: loop diuretics (furosemide), spironolactone
  - ACE inhibitors, angiotensin-receptor antagonists recommended; hydralazine and nitrates for those intolerant of these agents
  - Beta-blockers may exacerbate short-term symptoms; beneficial long-term
  - Digoxin improves symptoms in systolic failure
  - Dietary sodium and fluid restriction
  - Anticoagulation in normal sinus rhythm controversial
  - Dobutamine, milrinone, intra-aortic balloon pumps used in refractory cardiac failure as a bridge to surgery
  - Optimal management of diastolic heart failure: primarily beta-blockers and calcium-channel blockers

- **Pearl**

Symptomatic heart failure confers a worse prognosis than most cancers in the United States with a one-year mortality rate approaching 45%.

Reference

Liu P et al: The 2002/3 Canadian Cardiovascular Society consensus guideline update for the diagnosis and management of heart failure. Can J Cardiol 2003;19:347. [PMID: 12704478]

Heart Block

■ Essentials of Diagnosis
- Impaired conduction through atrioventricular (AV) node or bundle of His
- First-degree block: PR interval >210 msec; all atrial impulses conducted; asymptomatic
- Mobitz type I second-degree block (Wenckebach): PR interval lengthens with RR shortening before blocked beat; "grouped beating"; seen with inferior myocardial infarction; enhanced vagal tone
- Mobitz type II second-degree block: intermittent blocked beats without PR lengthening
- Third-degree block: complete AV dissociation; cannon a waves
- Fatigue, chest pain, dyspnea, dizziness, syncope when bradycardia associated with high-degree blocks (Mobitz II, third degree)
- Associated with myocardial injury, medications, myocarditis, infiltrative disorders (amyloid, sarcoid), electrolyte disturbances

■ Differential Diagnosis
- Sinus arrhythmia
- Atrial flutter
- Idioventricular rhythm
- Wandering pacemaker
- Atrial fibrillation
- Junctional rhythm
- AV dissociation
- Multifocal atrial tachycardia

■ Treatment
- Atropine treatment of choice for acute symptoms or severe bradycardia
- Blood pressure can be supported with dopamine or epinephrine
- Temporary pacing may be necessary: transcutaneous, transvenous
- Permanent pacemaker indicated in high-degree blocks
- Identify and treat underlying etiology: stop beta-blockers or AV blocking calcium channel blockers; reverse hyperkalemia
- Evaluate and manage ischemic cardiac disease

■ Pearl
AV dissociation and complete heart block are not synonymous. AV dissociation can occur without complete heart block when the intrinsic ventricular rate exceeds the sinus rate.

Reference

Brady WJ et al: Diagnosis and management of bradycardia and atrioventricular blocks associated with acute coronary ischemia. Emerg Med Clin North Am 2001;19:371. [PMID: 11373984]

Hypertensive Crisis & Malignant Hypertension

■ Essentials of Diagnosis

- Hypertensive crisis: blood pressure >240/130 or hypertension with comorbid condition requiring urgent control: angina, heart failure, cerebral hemorrhage, edema
- Malignant hypertension: severe hypertension with end-organ damage such as papilledema, encephalopathy, renal failure
- Irritability, headache, visual changes, nausea, confusion, chest pain, seizures
- Tachycardia, retinal hemorrhage or exudates, neurologic deficits
- Azotemia, disseminated intravascular coagulation
- Hematuria, red cell casts, proteinuria
- ECG: left ventricular hypertrophy, ischemic changes

■ Differential Diagnosis

- Accelerated essential hypertension
- Renovascular disease: renal artery stenosis
- Pheochromocytoma
- Acute glomerulonephritis
- Collagen vascular disease
- Food/drug interaction with monoamine oxidase inhibitor

■ Treatment

- Rapid reduction of blood pressure with short-acting titratable agents: nitroprusside, labetalol, esmolol, nitroglycerin
- Nitroprusside drug of choice; monitor thiocyanate levels after 24 hours of infusion especially in renal failure
- Labetalol or esmolol drip: utilize with underlying coronary artery disease
- ACE inhibitors: use in heart failure, myocardial infarction
- Nitroglycerin: primarily venodilator; variable blood pressure reduction; indicated for myocardial ischemia and heart failure
- Hydralazine: used as bridge from intravenous to oral medications
- Phentolamine preferred if pheochromocytoma suspected
- Hemodialysis can help with blood pressure control
- Assess degree of end-organ damage based on symptoms: head CT, renal ultrasound, echocardiogram

■ Pearl

Overly aggressive blood pressure reduction, especially in the case of an acute stroke, may lead to further cerebral ischemia and infarction secondary to impaired cerebral autoregulation.

Reference

Phillips RA et al: Hypertensive emergencies: diagnosis and management. Prog Cardiovasc Dis 2002;45:33. [PMID: 12138413]

Mesenteric Ischemia and Infarction, Acute

- **Essentials of Diagnosis**
  - Severe acute abdominal pain out of proportion to physical exam findings
  - Anorexia, nausea, vomiting, diarrhea, distention
  - Progression of ischemia and perforation leads to peritonitis, sepsis, shock, confusion
  - Leukocytosis, increased CK and LDH, severe metabolic acidosis, hyperamylasemia
  - Radiographs reveal air-fluid levels, dilated and thickened loops of bowel, pneumatosis intestinalis, perforation
  - "Thumbprinting" signs on barium contrast studies
  - Abdominal CT and angiography can be diagnostic
  - Risk factors: advanced age, cardiovascular disease, atherosclerosis, hypercoagulable states, malignancy, portal hypertension, systemic disorders, inflammation, trauma

- **Differential Diagnosis**
  - Pancreatitis
  - Appendicitis
  - Inflammatory bowel diseases
  - Cholecystitis and cholangitis
  - Peptic ulcer disease with or without perforation
  - Aortic dissection and ruptured aneurysms
  - Gynecologic pathologies
  - Diverticulitis
  - Vasculitis
  - Renal colic
  - Abdominal trauma

- **Treatment**
  - Aggressive fluid resuscitation
  - Maintain perfusion pressures; minimize vasopressor use
  - Correct electrolyte and acid-base disturbances
  - Broad-spectrum antibiotics covering enteric flora
  - Anticoagulation with heparin if not contraindicated
  - Angiographic evaluation if hemodynamically stable
  - Intra-arterial infusion of papaverine if emboli identified; utilized pre- and postoperatively
  - Surgical intervention often indicated: diagnosis, restoration of blood flow, resection of necrotic bowel
  - Thrombolytic therapies with anecdotal success; often used in poor surgical candidates

- **Pearl**

Controlling cardiac arrhythmias with digoxin may worsen mesenteric ischemia as this drug may promote mesenteric vasoconstriction.

Reference

Trompeter M et al: Non-occlusive mesenteric ischemia: etiology, diagnosis, and interventional therapy. Eur Radiol 2002;12:1179. [PMID: 11976865]

Mitral Valvular Heart Disease

■ Essentials of Diagnosis

- Dyspnea, orthopnea, paroxysmal nocturnal dyspnea, cough
- Signs and symptoms differ between acute and chronic lesions
- Mitral stenosis (MS): low-pitched diastolic murmur, crisp S1, opening snap, sternal heave, may have hemoptysis; atrial fibrillation common; >90% due to rheumatic heart disease (only 50–70% report history of rheumatic fever)
- Mitral regurgitation (MR): pansystolic murmur radiating to axilla; due to leaflet problems (endocarditis, myxomatous degeneration, rheumatic fever) or other problems of chordae tendineae, papillary muscles, mitral annulus; acute MR (myocardial infarction with papillary muscle dysfunction or endocarditis)
- Echocardiogram essential in confirming and assessing diagnosis

■ Differential Diagnosis

- Mitral stenosis: left atrial myxoma, mitral valve prolapse, pulmonary hypertension, atrial septal defect
- Mitral regurgitation: aortic stenosis, hypertrophic cardiomyopathy, ventricular septal defect (VSD)

■ Treatment

- Mitral stenosis: slow heart rate maximizes left ventricular filling time, especially if atrial fibrillation (beta-blockers, digoxin, diltiazem); cardioversion; diuretics; no role of afterload reduction; balloon valvuloplasty; mitral valve replacement
- Mitral regurgitation: afterload reduction may help forward flow (ACE inhibitors, hydralazine plus nitrates, nitroprusside); diuretics; mitral valve replacement
- Infective endocarditis prophylaxis
- Cardiac catheterization often necessary prior to surgery
- Surgical valve repair or replacement ideally indicated for all symptomatic patients

■ Pearl

Acute mitral regurgitation may have sudden onset of pulmonary edema, hypotension, and shock; chronic mitral regurgitation may cause unexplained fatigue and exercise intolerance.

Reference

Bonow RO et al: ACC/AHA guidelines for the management of patients with valvular heart disease. J Am Coll Cardiol 1998;32:1486. [PMID: 9809971]

Myocardial Infarction (AMI), Acute

- **Essentials of Diagnosis**
  - Prolonged substernal chest pressure; lasting >15 minutes
  - Discomfort radiates to left arm, neck, or jaw; sweating, nausea, vomiting, syncope
  - Right ventricular MI: suspect with inferior MI or hypotension with nitrate administration; confirm with right-sided ECG
  - ECG with ST segment elevation (tombstones) >1 mm in two contiguous leads or new bundle branch block
  - Elevation of CK-MB, troponins, AST, LDH
  - Echocardiogram: identifies wall motion abnormalities, residual ventricular function, valvular abnormalities, MI associated tamponade
  - Complications: tachy/bradyarrhythmias, heart block, valvular insufficiencies, pulmonary edema, hypoxemia, cardiogenic shock, pericarditis

- **Differential Diagnosis**
  - Cardiovascular: stable or unstable angina, Prinzmetal angina, pericarditis, myocarditis, aortic dissection
  - Pulmonary: pneumothorax, pulmonary embolism, pneumonia
  - Gastrointestinal: esophageal reflux or spasm, gastritis, peptic ulcer disease, cholangitis, hepatitis, pancreatitis
  - Musculoskeletal pain and costochondritis

- **Treatment**
  - Bed rest, monitoring, oxygen, serial cardiac enzymes, ECGs
  - Immediately chew and swallow aspirin; clopidogrel in those intolerant of aspirin
  - Pain control with nitrates and/or morphine; anxiolytics
  - Beta-blockers to reduce myocardial oxygen consumption
  - ACE inhibitors confer survival benefit when EF < 40%,
  - Thrombolytic reperfusion in ST segment elevation or new left bundle branch block if no contraindication
  - Primary angioplasty alternative to thrombolytics if unstable hemodynamics or chest pain on optimal medical regimen
  - Right heart catheterization may aid management of hypotension

- **Pearl**

When an AMI is thought to be associated with cocaine use, the use of selective beta-blockers may lead to unopposed alpha-adrenergic stimulation and worsening hypertension and cardiac injury.

Reference

Cannon CP et al: Critical pathways for management of patients with acute coronary syndromes: an assessment by the National Heart Attack Alert Program. Am Heart J 2002;143:777. [PMID: 12040337]

Supraventricular Tachycardia

- ■ Essentials of Diagnosis
  - Tachycardia (heart rate >100) with origin of electrical rhythm within atria or atrioventricular (AV) node resulting in narrow QRS complex (<120 msec)
  - Palpitations, dyspnea, chest pain
  - ECG and rhythm strip essential for diagnosis
  - Constant rate as clue to arrhythmia: 150 consider atrial flutter with 2:1 block; 180 consider AV nodal reentry
  - Regularity can guide differential diagnosis: regular (ST, AVNRT, AVRT, AT, JT), irregular (MFAT, A-fib), either (A-flut)
  - MFAT often associated with severe lung disease
  - Suspect accessory tract if PR interval shortened and ventricular rate >200; examine rhythm strip for delta waves

- ■ Differential Diagnosis
  - Sinus tachycardia (ST)
  - AV nodal reentry tachycardia (AVNRT)
  - Atrioventricular reentry via accessory pathway (AVRT)
  - Ectopic atrial tachycardia (AT)
  - Multifocal atrial tachycardia (MFAT)
  - Junctional tachycardia (JT)
  - Atrial flutter (A-flut)
  - Atrial fibrillation (A-fib)

- ■ Treatment
  - Adenosine to evaluate underlying rhythm; often terminates AVNRT; uncovers fibrillatory and flutter waves
  - AV nodal blockade and rate control
  - Urgent electrical cardioversion when hemodynamically unstable
  - Reverse potential precipitating factors: electrolytes, hypoxemia, alkalosis, ischemia
  - Antiarrhythmics useful in A-fib, A-flut, AT
  - Overdrive atrial pacing can be attempted
  - Electrophysiological study in refractory cases with or without ablation

- ■ Pearl

In patients with supraventricular tachycardia and evidence of an accessory bypass tract (Wolff-Parkinson-White syndrome), the use of AV nodal blocking agents should be avoided as they can promote antegrade accessory pathway conduction and worsen tachycardia. Procainamide is the agent of choice.

Reference

Blomstrom-Lundquist C et al: ACC/AHA/ESC guidelines for the management of patients with supraventricular arrhythmias. J Am Coll Cardiol 2003 Oct 15;42:1493. [PMID: 14563598]

Syncope

- ■ Essentials of Diagnosis
  - Transient loss of consciousness and postural tone with prompt recovery
  - Pallor and generalized perspiration prior to event
  - Cardiac syncope: chest discomfort, dyspnea, palpitations
  - Vasovagal syncope: prodrome of light-headedness, diaphoresis, nausea, "aura"
  - Bradycardia and hypotension not always identified
  - Monitor ECG and rhythm strip
  - Echocardiogram to identify structural heart disease
  - Tilt-table testing to evaluate vasovagal symptoms

- ■ Differential Diagnosis
  - Cardiovascular: arrhythmias, outflow tract obstruction
  - Pulmonary vascular disease: pulmonary embolism, pulmonary hypertension
  - Vasovagal syndrome and situational syncope: cough, micturition, pain
  - Postural hypotension and autonomic dysfunction
  - Neurologic: cerebrovascular accidents, vertebrobasilar insufficiency, seizures
  - Metabolic derangements: hypoglycemia
  - Hypoxemia
  - Hysterical fainting

- ■ Treatment
  - Identify and correct underlying etiology
  - When patient is unconscious, position horizontally and secure airway
  - In vasovagal syncope effective prophylaxis can be achieved with beta-blockers; theophylline, scopolamine, disopyramide, ephedrine, support stockings tried with varying success
  - Pacemakers: adjunct in management of cardioinhibitory responses seen in vasovagal syndromes; indicated in bradyarrhythmias
  - Fludrocortisone helpful in autonomic dysfunction
  - Electrophysiology studies and implantable defibrillators can be considered in tachyarrhythmias especially ventricular in origin
  - Advise against driving

- ■ Pearl

In tilt-table testing for vasovagal syndromes, vasodepressor and cardioinhibitory responses may be seen but are diagnostic only when associated with symptoms.

Reference

Kapoor WN et al: Current evaluation and management of syncope. Circulation 2002;106:1606. [PMID: 12270849]

Unstable Angina (USA) & Non–ST–Segment Elevation Myocardial Infarction (NSTEMI)

- **Essentials of Diagnosis**
  - Heavy, pressure-like substernal chest discomfort with radiation to neck, jaw, left arm; nausea, diaphoresis, dyspnea
  - Complications: arrhythmia, hypotension, pulmonary edema
  - ECG may reveal ≥ 1 mm ST segment depression or T wave inversion
  - Elevated cardiac enzymes (troponin, CK-MB) indicate myocardial necrosis

- **Differential Diagnosis**
  - Angina pectoris, Prinzmetal angina, pericarditis, myocarditis, aortic dissection
  - Pneumothorax, pulmonary embolism, pneumonia
  - Reflux esophagitis, esophageal spasm, gastritis, pancreatitis
  - Musculoskeletal pain and costochondritis

- **Treatment**
  - Bed rest, oxygen, monitoring, serial cardiac enzymes
  - Initiate aspirin and continue indefinitely
  - Beta-blockers for heart rate and blood pressure control; nondihydropyridine calcium antagonists if beta-blockers contraindicated
  - Nitrates for relief of symptoms
  - Morphine for persistent pain or pulmonary edema
  - ACE inhibitors when hypertension persists: especially if EF $< 40\%$ or if diabetic
  - HMG-CoA reductase inhibitors with goal LDL < 100
  - Clopidogrel for those intolerable of aspirin or as adjunct for percutaneous coronary intervention (PCI)
  - Unfractionated or low-molecular-weight heparin with benefits
  - Platelet glycoprotein IIb/IIIa antagonists if PCI planned
  - Early PCI for high-risk patients: recurrent symptoms on medications, congestive heart failure, ventricular arrhythmia, unstable hemodynamics, elevated troponin

- **Pearl**

A minority of patients with normal coronary arteries may present with USA due to increased workload on the heart: anemia, thyrotoxicosis, hypoxemia, hypotension.

Reference

Braunwald E et al: ACC/AHA 2002 guideline update for the management of patients with unstable angina and non-ST-segment elevation myocardial infarction. J Am Coll Cardiol 2002;40:1366. [PMID: 12383588]

Ventricular Tachyarrhythmias

- **Essentials of Diagnosis**
  - More than three consecutive ventricular beats or broad-complex tachycardia with rate >100 and QRS >120 msec; "sustained" if ventricular tachycardia (VT) lasts >30 seconds
  - Chest pain, dyspnea, flushing, palpitations, dizziness, syncope, sudden death
  - Torsade de pointes associated with prolonged QT; can degenerate into ventricular fibrillation (VF)
  - ECG and rhythm strip key to diagnosis
  - Features highly suggestive of VT: AV dissociation, fusion beats, concordance of QRS, failure to slow down with adenosine, extreme right or left axis deviation
  - Etiologies: ischemia, cardiomyopathy, valvular heart disease, antiarrhythmics, sympathomimetics, electrolyte disturbances, drugs that prolong QT interval, mechanical irritation (central lines)

- **Differential Diagnosis**
  - Preexisting conduction defect (bundle branch block, BBB) with supraventricular tachyarrhythmia (SVT)
  - SVT with aberrant conduction
  - Antegrade conduction through an accessory pathway

- **Treatment**
  - Immediate cardioversion when hemodynamically compromised
  - Adenosine if unclear if VT or SVT
  - Treat correctable underlying factors
  - Evaluate potential ischemic cardiac disease
  - Acute antiarrhythmics unnecessary if episode brief and self-terminating
  - Consider antiarrhythmics when episode prolonged especially if hemodynamic changes or underlying myocardial disease: lidocaine, procainamide, amiodarone
  - May use beta-blockers in setting of high catecholamine state
  - In VF and pulseless VT: amiodarone and procainamide
  - Magnesium drug of choice in torsade de pointes

- **Pearl**

All antiarrhythmic agents can be proarrhythmic. Thus, the use of these agents in asymptomatic individuals with episodic premature ventricular contractions may carry a higher risk than benefit profile.

Reference

Hohnloser SH et al: Changing late prognosis of acute myocardial infarction: Impact on management of ventricular arrhythmias. Circulation 2003;107:941. [PMID: 12600904]

Botulism

Diagnosis

ending paralysis caused by neurotoxin produced by
botulinum; at least three of nausea, vomiting, dys-
opia, dilated fixed pupils, dry mouth in 90%
ves affected first, followed by descending symmet-
paralysis, respiratory muscle involvement slowly or
ressive
disturbances, changes in sensorium, fever; cranial
pared
detection of toxin in serum, stool, vomitus, gastric
ected food
al forms: (1) food-borne from ingestion of pre-
(onset 2 hours to 8 days); (2) wound with toxin
infection with *C botulinum* (rare, incubation period
en with cutaneous illicit drug use); (3) in infants,
botulism spores, which germinate in the gut and
s
rsibly blocks acetylcholine release at peripheral
r junctions leading to flaccid paralysis

nosis

avis and Eaton-Lambert syndrome

syndrome (Miller-Fisher variant)

e with frequent monitoring of vital capacity to
ory failure; intubation, mechanical ventilation
um antitoxin (trivalent or polyvalent); patients
for hypersensitivity
devitalized tissue for wound botulism; penicillin
ction
ecrease GI colonization with *C botulinum* con-

*er develops descending paralysis, suspect wound
black tar heroin."*

ent of botulism. Ann Pharmacother 2003;37:127.

10

Infectious Disease

Ba

- **Essentials of Diagno**
  - Acute-onset fever,
    may have vomitin
    tures of sepsis (h
    nated intravascula
    techial or ecchyn
  - Purulent cerebros
    neutrophil predc
    (<50% of serum
    of fluid
  - Culture of bactei
    diagnosis
  - In adults, *S pn*
    gram-negative b
    rosurgical proce

- **Differential Diagn**
  - Viral, fungal,
  - Carcinomatous
  - Drug-induced

- **Treatment**
  - Supportive ca
    respiratory fai
  - Third-generat
  - Add ampicilli
    for suspected

- **Pearl**

Look for an infecti
toiditis, sinusitis,
cal drainage.

Reference

Beaman MH: Acut
  Aust 2002;176:3

- **Essentials o**
  - Acute des
    Clostridiu
    phagia, di
  - Cranial ne
    rical flacci
    rapidly pro
  - No sensor
    nerves I, II
  - Confirm by
    aspirate, su
  - Three clini
    formed tox
    produced by
    4–14 days,
    ingestion of
    produce tox
  - Toxin irrev
    neuromuscu

- **Differential Dia**
  - Myasthenia
  - Tick paralys
  - Poliomyelitis
  - Guillain-Bar
  - Stroke
  - Rabies
  - Diphtheria

- **Treatment**
  - Supportive c
    predict respir
  - Equine botuli
    must be teste
  - Debridement
    for wound inf
  - Antibiotics to
    troversial

- **Pearl**

If an injection drug u
botulism caused by

Reference

Robinson RF: Manage
  [PMID: 12503947].

Central Nervous System (CNS) Infections in HIV-Infected Patients

- **Essentials of Diagnosis**

  - Cryptococcal meningitis: headache and/or fever dominant findings, India ink test on CSF—sensitivity 70%; CSF cryptococcal antigen >95% sensitive; CSF culture >98% sensitive
  - Toxoplasmosis: focal neurologic deficits common; CT scan: >2 ring-enhancing lesions involving basal ganglia; serum toxoplasma antibody in >95%; primary CNS lymphoma usually single large lesion in deep periventricular space with variable enhancement
  - PML: cognitive deficits common; multiple hypodense lesions in white matter on MRI, usually without edema or enhancement; JC virus CSF PCR 80% sensitive; distinguish from HIV dementia and encephalopathy

- **Differential Diagnosis**

  - Noninfectious HIV-associated neurologic disorders: HIV dementia and encephalopathy, primary CNS lymphoma
  - Stroke
  - Primary or metastatic brain tumor

- **Treatment**

  - CNS toxoplasmosis: sulfadiazine plus pyrimethamine and leucovorin; empiric therapy for suspected cases pending results of serum toxoplasma antibody; reevaluate clinical and radiographic response (MRI or CT) in 7–10 days
  - Cryptococcal meningitis: Amphotericin B + 5-flucytosine followed by fluconazole
  - Secondary prophylaxis indicated for toxoplasmosis and cryptococcal meningitis
  - PML and HIV dementia: no specific therapy available; antiretroviral therapy associated with improved outcome
  - Consider optimal timing of antiretroviral therapy to avoid immune reconstitution syndrome (toxoplasmosis, tuberculous meningitis, PML)

- **Pearl**

  Meningismus is rare in cryptococcal meningitis, and CSF profile may be completely normal.

Reference

Ammassari A: Diagnosis of AIDS-related focal brain lesions: a decision-making analysis based on clinical and neuroradiologic characteristics combined with polymerase chain reaction assays in CSF. Neurology 1997;48:687. [PMID: 9065549]

Clostridium difficile-Associated Diarrhea

- **Essentials of Diagnosis**
  - Ranges from simple diarrhea to pseudomembranous colitis; rarely megacolon, perforation and death
  - Low-grade fever, leukocytosis common; abdominal pain rare in uncomplicated cases
  - Occurs in patients colonized with *C difficile*, when selective antibiotic pressure induces toxin production; frequency of colonization increases with duration of hospitalization (20% colonized at 1 week, 50% at 1 month); may occur after single dose of antibiotic, up to 6 weeks after antibiotic
  - *C difficile* produces two toxins (toxin A, enterotoxin; toxin B, cytotoxin); send stool for toxin assay; repeat increases diagnostic yield
  - Ampicillin, clindamycin and cephalosporins most frequently associated; trimethoprim-sulfamethoxazole, quinolones, aztreonam, carbapenems, metronidazole rarely

- **Differential Diagnosis**
  - Noninfectious diarrhea (ischemic colitis, inflammatory bowel disease, gastrointestinal bleeding)
  - Antibiotic-associated diarrhea (not *C difficile*-induced)
  - Enteric pathogens (rare in ICU)

- **Treatment**
  - Discontinue toxin-inducing antibiotics
  - Oral metronidazole
  - Oral vancomycin more expensive, associated with risk of vancomycin-resistant enterococci
  - 20% relapse within 2 weeks; retreat with metronidazole; increased risk of relapse if prior *C difficile* diarrhea, continuation of inducing antibiotics, community-acquisition, significant leukocytosis
  - Asymptomatic *C difficile* carriage should not be treated (prolongs carrier stage)

- **Pearl**

C difficile can survive on environmental surfaces (medical devices, countertops); use precautions to prevent nosocomial transmission.

Reference

Mylonakis E: *Clostridium difficile*-associated diarrhea: a review. Arch Intern Med 2001;161:525. [PMID: 11252111]

Community-Acquired Pneumonia

- **Essentials of Diagnosis**
  - Acute onset of fever, productive cough, respiratory distress; sometimes chills, occasional pleuritic chest pain; fever, tachypnea, hypoxemia
  - Chest radiograph with patchy, localized infiltrates or consolidation; may be bilateral, diffuse
  - Mortality 5–36%; higher if male, diabetes mellitus, neurologic or neoplastic disease, hypothermia, hypotension, leukopenia, multilobar infiltrates, bacteremia, advanced age, resistant organism
  - *Streptococcus pneumoniae* most common pathogen identified followed by *Haemophilus influenzae*; aerobic gram-negative bacilli uncommon except in alcoholics, nursing home residents; *Chlamydia pneumoniae*, *Mycoplasma pneumoniae* typically cause milder pneumonia
  - Suspect legionella, if outbreak; tuberculosis, endemic mycosis (*C immitis*, *H capsulatum*), if relevant exposure; *Pneumocystis carinii* (*jiroveci*), if HIV risk

- **Differential Diagnosis**
  - Pulmonary edema
  - Pulmonary hemorrhage
  - Hypersensitivity pneumonitis
  - Lung cancer
  - Chemical pneumonitis

- **Treatment**
  - Manage respiratory failure, hypotension
  - Obtain sputum Gram stain, blood cultures
  - Early antibiotics improve outcome
  - For most patients, third-generation cephalosporin plus macrolide or doxycycline, or fluoroquinolone with antipneumococcal activity (levofloxacin) alone
  - Consider broader antibiotic coverage if patient diabetic, alcoholic

- **Pearl**

Pneumonia caused by penicillin-resistant Streptococcus pneumoniae (except very highly resistant strains) is effectively treated with usual antibiotics; however, vancomycin should be added if meningitis suspected.

Reference

Bartlett JG: Practice guidelines for management of community-acquired pneumonia in adults. Clin Infect Dis 2000;31:347. [PMID: 10987697]

Encephalitis, Brain Abscess, Spinal Epidural Abscess

- **Essentials of Diagnosis**
  - Encephalitis: altered sensorium, headache, fever, sometimes progressing to stupor, coma, occasionally seizures, focal neurologic signs; Herpes simplex most common sporadic viral encephalitis; arboviruses, West Nile virus
  - Brain abscess: fever, seizures, focal neurologic signs, progressive obtundation; abnormal head CT (with radiographic contrast) or MRI; may have local infection (otitis media, sinusitis, dental infection)
  - Spinal epidural abscess: fever, back pain, radiculopathy, progressive motor or sensory deficits depending on location, percussion tenderness; may have adjacent osteomyelitis

- **Differential Diagnosis**
  - CNS tumor (primary or metastatic to spine or brain)
  - Bacterial or viral meninigitis
  - Fungal or tuberculous infection, especially in immunocompromised host
  - Vasculitis or collagen vascular diseases

- **Treatment**
  - Evaluate for CNS or spinal cord mass effect or compression
  - High-dose acyclovir for herpes encephalitis
  - Surgical drainage for spinal epidural abscess
  - Antibiotics for epidural abscess active against staphylococci, streptococci, gram-negative bacilli; for brain abscess active against streptococci plus anaerobes

- **Pearl**

Brain abscesses arising from the oral cavity and frontal or ethmoid sinuses tend to locate in the frontal lobes of the brain; hematologically seeded abscesses are more often multiple and occur in the area supplied by the middle cerebral artery.

Reference

Beaman MH: Acute community-acquired meningitis and encephalitis. Med J Aust 2002;176:389. [PMID: 12041637]

Fever in the ICU

- **Essentials of Diagnosis**
  - Temperature >38.3°C orally or rectally; axillary temperature measurements not accurate
  - In critically ill, both noninfectious and infectious etiologies must be considered, including drug reactions
  - Evaluate based on underlying medical conditions, symptoms and signs, recent infections, current or recent antibiotics, review of medication record, laboratory findings

- **Differential Diagnosis**
  - Infectious causes: sepsis, pneumonia, urinary tract infection (especially if indwelling urinary catheter), intravenous catheter infection (with or without signs of inflammation at insertion site), *Clostridium difficile* colitis, infected decubitus ulcer, sinusitis (especially with nasotracheal or nasogastric tube), intra-abdominal infections, endocarditis
  - Noninfectious causes of fever include drugs or allergic reactions, deep venous thrombosis, central nervous system fever, intraventricular hemorrhage, tissue necrosis, malignancy, hyperthyroidism, neuroleptic-malignant syndrome

- **Treatment**
  - Specific treatment determined by etiology of fever
  - Empiric antibiotic therapy if high suspicion for infection; obtain cultures prior to initiating antibiotics
  - Administer antipyretics; consider physical cooling (ice packs, cooling blanket, cool fluids, intravenously or via peritoneum, cold hemodialysis) if severe hyperthermia

- **Pearl**

Antibiotic treatment of colonized sites unnecessary, and likely to select for resistant organisms.

Reference

Cunha BA: Fever in the intensive care unit. Intensive Care Med 1999;25:648. [PMID:10470566]

Hematogenously Disseminated Candidiasis

- **Essentials of Diagnosis**
  - Persistent fever despite broad-spectrum antibiotics; may be complicated by candida endocarditis, osteomyelitis, arthritis, hepatosplenic candidiasis, endophthalmitis, CNS abscesses
  - Risk factors: number of antimicrobial agents given, duration of antimicrobial therapy, total parenteral nutrition, neutropenia, hemodialysis, colonization with candida, extensive surgeries, burns
  - Candida fourth leading organism isolated from blood cultures in hospitalized patients; however, sensitivity of blood cultures for detecting candidemia <50%
  - *C albicans* most common species isolated (59%); but increasing isolation of nonalbicans species, especially *C glabrata*

- **Differential Diagnosis**
  - Noninfectious source of persistent fever (DVT, drug fever, embolic events)
  - Other infectious causes of fever (bacteria, mycobacteria, viruses, other fungi)

- **Treatment**
  - Empiric antifungal therapy in patients with persistent fever and significant risk factors
  - Antifungal agent selected depends on knowledge of *Candida* spp and patient's status
  - Amphotericin B standard treatment; consider fluconazole in non-neutropenic patients with susceptible *Candida* spp
  - Role of newer antifungal agents in candida bloodstream infection under investigation
  - Removal of indwelling catheters strongly advised

- **Pearl**

Presence of endophthalmitis must be excluded in patients with candidemia; if found, prolonged systemic therapy, and, in advanced cases, vitrectomy required.

Reference

Spellberg B: The pathophysiology and treatment of candida sepsis. Curr Infect Dis Rep 2002;5:387. [PMID: 12228025]

Infections in Immunocompromised Hosts

- **Essentials of Diagnosis**
  - Suspected infection in patients with immunocompromising condition, such as neutropenia, organ transplantation with immunosuppressive therapy, diabetes, splenectomy, chronic corticosteroid therapy, HIV infection; type of immunocompromise determines risk, nature of opportunistic infection
  - Neutropenia associated with gram-negative bacilli, gram-positive cocci, fungi
  - Organ transplant recipients susceptible to *Pneumocystis jiroveci*, *Listeria monocytogenes*, *Nocardia asteroides*, *Cryptococcus neoformans*, *Aspergillus* spp, cytomegalovirus (2–6 months after transplant)
  - Postsplenectomy: overwhelming infection with encapsulated organisms, such as *S pneumoniae*, *N meningitides*, *H influenzae*
  - Diabetics prone to more severe manifestations of common infections (emphysematous cholecystitis and pyelonephritis, necrotizing soft tissue infection) plus specific infections (rhinocerebral mucormycosis, malignant otitis externa)

- **Treatment**
  - Antimicrobial therapy against likely organisms based on immunocompromising condition, specific clinical features
  - Surgical debridement for emphysematous infections, infections with necrosis, rhinocerebral mucormycosis
  - Vaccination against *S pneumoniae*, *H influenzae* and *N meningitidis* in asplenic and HIV-infected patients, others at increased risk

- **Pearl**

A functional asplenic state can occur in congenital hyposplenism, sickle cell disease, graft-versus-host disease, rheumatoid arthritis, systemic lupus erythematosus, amyloidosis, ulcerative colitis, celiac disease, and chronic alcoholism.

Reference

Fishman JA: Infection in organ-transplant recipients. N Engl J Med 1998;338:1741. [PMID: 9624195]

Infective Endocarditis

- ■ **Essentials of Diagnosis**
  - • Presentation depends on infecting organism
  - • Acute staphylococcal endocarditis: short prodrome, sepsis syndrome; viridans streptococci: classical subacute endocarditis with murmur, conjunctival hemorrhage, Janeway lesions, immunologic phenomena (Roth spots, Osler nodes, immune complex glomerulonephritis)
  - • Diagnosis by Duke criteria: major (positive blood cultures or typical findings on echocardiography) plus minor (vascular and immunologic phenomenon, echocardiography and blood culture results not meeting major), fever, predisposing factors
  - • Risk factors: underlying valvular abnormality, prosthetic valves, injection drug use
  - • Common organisms: *S aureus* (~50%; injection drug users and diabetics), viridans streptococci, enterococci; less common pathogens *S pneumoniae*, group A, B, C streptococci, *L monocytogenes*, *P aeruginosa*, *S marcescens*
  - • If blood cultures negative, consider "HACEK" group (*Haemophilus*, *Actinobacillus*, *Cardiobacterium*, *Eikenella*, *Kingella*), and *Brucella*, *Legionella*, *Bartonella*, *Coxiella*, fungi
  - • Transesophageal echocardiography preferred imaging study

- ■ **Differential Diagnosis**
  - • Bacteremia from other sites
  - • Marantic endocarditis
  - • Atrial myxoma
  - • Thrombophlebitis
  - • Rheumatic diseases

- ■ **Treatment**
  - • Systemic antibiotic directed against causative organism for 4–6 weeks; consider 2 weeks of combination therapy for uncomplicated right sided endocarditis in selected patients
  - • Surgical valve replacement for failure of medical therapy, decompensated CHF from valvular insufficiency, continued septic emboli despite antibiotic therapy, fungal endocarditis

- ■ **Pearl**

Consider endocarditis in every patient presenting with fever and stroke.

Reference

DiNubile MJ: Infective endocarditis. N Engl J Med 2002;346:782. [PMID: 11882739]

Intra-abdominal Infection

- **Essentials of Diagnosis**
  - Wide array of clinical syndromes, including intraperitoneal, pancreatic and hepatic abscesses, spontaneous and secondary peritonitis, colitis, cholangitis
  - Symptoms often nonspecific, such as vague abdominal pain, anorexia, fever
  - Bowel sounds may be diminished or absent
  - Laboratory findings nonspecific
  - Abdominal imaging by CT scan (abscess or perforation) or ultrasound (biliary process) useful to localize site of infection
  - Majority of infections are polymicrobial, involving native gastrointestinal flora (aerobic and microaerophilic streptococci, enterobacteriaceae, enterococci and anaerobes); hepatic abscess from *Entamoeba histolytica*
  - GI colonization with *Candida* spp in about 50% of patients
  - Antibiotic use increases likelihood of *Candida* spp, resistant gram-negative bacilli, enterococci

- **Differential Diagnosis**
  - Ischemic bowel
  - Perforated viscus, pancreatitis, peptic ulcer disease, biliary colic
  - Tumors

- **Treatment**
  - Broad-spectrum antimicrobial therapy targeting enteric flora (especially gram-negative bacilli and anaerobes)
  - Antifungal therapy in patients with significant risk factors
  - Surgical drainage of abscesses and debridement of necrotic tissue

- **Pearl**

Lack of physical findings in intra-abdominal infection is common in immunocompromised (steroids, chemotherapy, neutropenia), obese, and elderly patients.

Reference

McClean KL: Intraabdominal infection: a review. Clin Infect Dis 1994;19:100.
 [PMID: 7948510]

Intravenous Catheter-Associated Infection

- **Essentials of Diagnosis**
  - Local infection at catheter exit site with erythema, purulence, tenderness up to 2 cm from insertion site
  - Tunnel infection has signs of infection >2 cm from skin insertion site
  - Catheter-associated sepsis caused by migration of skin-colonizing organism to tip of catheter, contamination of catheter hub, or rarely hematogenous seeding of catheter or infusion of contaminated fluids
  - Catheter-associated bloodstream infection when same organism grown from catheter tip and blood cultures
  - Gram-positive organisms most common (coagulase negative staphylococci, *Staphylococcus aureus*), but increasing incidence of candida, gram-negative organisms (associated with monitoring devices and contaminated intravenous fluids)
  - No agreement on quantitative and semiquantitative cultures for diagnosis; some define infection as >15 colony-forming units or >10^3 organism cultured from distal catheter tip

- **Differential Diagnosis**
  - Chemical phlebitis
  - Thrombophlebitis or thrombosis of central venous catheter
  - Bacteremia, sepsis from noncatheter source

- **Treatment**
  - Remove catheter whenever possible; removal strongly indicated in presence of sepsis, or if resistant or difficult to treat pathogen isolated (fungi, *Pseudomonas aeruginosa*)
  - Antibiotic therapy against most likely pathogens (empiric vancomycin plus aminoglycoside or cephalosporin is appropriate)

- **Pearl**

To minimize risk of infection, always use a new insertion site for replacement of an intravenous catheter.

Reference

Cunha BA: Intravenous line infections. Crit Care Clin 1998;14:339. [PMID: 9561821]

Mycobacterium tuberculosis

- **Essentials of Diagnosis**
  - Fever, night sweats, weight loss, fatigue, productive cough; sometimes hemoptysis
  - Upper lobe infiltrate most common (posterior and apical segments), if reactivation; primary TB involves lower lobes; chest radiograph may be normal in presence of HIV infection
  - Acid-fast smear; tuberculosis cultured from sputum; positive cultures from blood and urine in disseminated disease; if localized to lymph nodes, may require biopsy for diagnosis
  - TB skin test (PPD) may be nonreactive in critically ill patients
  - Pulmonary tuberculosis most common syndrome in adults; adenitis in children
  - Increased tuberculosis incidence in HIV-infected persons, homeless, foreign-born, institutionalized patients; high mortality (>50%) if respiratory failure
  - Susceptibility testing recommended in all cases to identify drug-resistant strains

- **Differential Diagnosis**
  - Bacterial pneumonia
  - Malignancy
  - Fungal pneumonia (cocidioidomycosis, histoplasmosis)
  - Pulmonary emboli
  - Pneumocystis pneumonia in HIV-positive patients
  - Lung abscess

- **Treatment**
  - Respiratory isolation for all suspected patients
  - Manage respiratory failure
  - If no prior treatment, isoniazid (INH), rifampin, pyrazinamide, ethambutol for 2 months; followed by INH and rifampin for at least 4 months; directly observed treatment (DOT) strongly recommended
  - If prior treatment for tuberculosis, expert consultation recommended; if resistant mycobacteria isolated, modify therapy according to susceptibility testing

- **Pearl**

In the presence of a positive TB skin test, risk for developing active tuberculosis is 10% during lifetime in immunocompetent patients, but 10% per year in patients with HIV infection.

Reference

Lee PL: Patient mortality of active pulmonary tuberculosis requiring mechanical ventilation. Eur Respir J 2003;22:141. [PMID: 12882464]

Necrotizing Soft Tissue Infection

- ■ Essentials of Diagnosis
  - Rapidly spreading infection with widespread tissue necrosis with potentially high mortality rate
  - Clinical features disproportionate to physical findings; edema and tenderness beyond area of erythema, palpable crepitus, vesicles or bullae
  - Fever, tachycardia, hypotension common
  - Leukocytosis, disseminated intravascular coagulation, elevated creatinine kinase, acidosis, renal failure
  - Three types: Group A streptococcal infection; clostridial infection (gas gangrene, myonecrosis); polymicrobial infection (eg, Fournier disease)
  - Patients with impaired host defense at higher risk

- ■ Differential Diagnosis
  - Cellulitis
  - Myositis
  - Thrombophlebitis
  - Compartment syndrome
  - Soft tissue abscess

- ■ Treatment
  - Early diagnosis and aggressive treatment critical for survival
  - Emergent surgical exploration indicated for any suspicion of necrotizing soft tissue infection
  - Immediate surgical exploration and debridement; surgical reexploration every 1–2 days to ensure that wound edges are free of necrosis
  - Broad-spectrum antibiotics to cover aerobic and anaerobic organisms

- ■ Pearl

Findings suggestive of invasive soft tissue involvement, such as crepitus or blistering, are present in <40% of patients.

Reference

Nichols RL: Clinical presentations of soft-tissue infections and surgical site infections. Clin Infect Dis 2001;33(Suppl 2):S84. [PMID: 11486304]

Neutropenic Fever

- **Essentials of Diagnosis**
  - Single temperature >38.3°C, or ≥38°C for 1 hour, in patient with neutropenia (absolute neutrophil count <500/μL, or <1000/μL with anticipated decline to <500/μL)
  - Up to 90% of neutropenic patients develop fever
  - Duration, depth, cause of neutropenia determine likelihood of infection; infection most common cause of death during neutropenic episodes
  - Common pathogens include aerobic gram-negative bacilli, with increasing incidence of gram-positive cocci; but etiology identified in only 30–50%; only 10–20% have documented bacteremia or fungemia
  - Fever often only sign of infection; however, complete history and careful examination essential (inspect skin, mucous membranes, perirectal area)

- **Differential Diagnosis**
  - Drug fever or allergic reaction
  - Fever secondary to hematologic malignancy
  - Deep venous thrombosis

- **Treatment**
  - Prompt initiation of empiric antimicrobial therapy using antipseudomonal beta-lactam antibiotic with or without aminoglycoside
  - Add antistaphylococcal/streptococcal agent (vancomycin) in patients at higher risk for gram-positive cocci (central IV catheter, mucositis, prior treatment with fluoroquinolones)
  - Antifungal agents indicated in prolonged neutropenic fever (>5 days) despite broad-spectrum antibacterial drugs
  - Avoid rectal exams, which can lead to bacteremia

- **Pearl**

Physical exam may be misleading because lack of neutrophils precludes usual pus formation, fluctuance, or development of abscesses.

Reference

Hughes WT: 2002 guidelines for the use of antimicrobial agents in neutropenic patients with cancer. Clin Infect Dis 2002;34:730. [PMID: 11850858]

Nonbacterial Meningitis

- **Essentials of Diagnosis**
    - Acute onset of headache, mild neck stiffness, fever (viral meningitis); chronic symptoms with gradual increase in severity over days to weeks (tuberculous or fungal meningitis)
    - May have features of underlying disease (viral syndrome or pulmonary or disseminated tuberculosis or fungal infection)
    - Viral meningitis: acute onset, resolves within days; cerebrospinal fluid with predominance of lymphocytes, normal glucose; enteroviruses most commonly implicated
    - Tuberculous meningitis: subacute or chronic onset of symptoms; cerebrospinal fluid with predominance of lymphocytes, low glucose, high protein
    - Fungal meningitis: subacute or chronic onset of symptoms; cerebrospinal fluid has predominance of lymphocytes; variably low glucose and high protein (*Coccidioides immitis*); in *Cryptococcus neoformans* meningitis, symptoms, signs often unremarkable; may have high CSF opening pressure and positive CSF India ink stain, but normal glucose, protein, cell counts

- **Differential Diagnosis**
    - Carcinomatous meningitis
    - Partially treated bacterial meningitis
    - Drug-induced meningitis

- **Treatment**
    - No specific treatment for viral meningitis
    - Tuberculous meningitis: begin empiric therapy with 3–4 antituberculous drugs
    - Cryptococcal meningitis: amphotericin B plus 5-flucytosine followed by fluconazole
    - Coccidioides meningitis: high dose fluconazole, or fluconazole + amphotericin B

- **Pearl**

Mumps, Herpes simplex, and lymphochoriomeningitis (LCM) meningoencephalitis may cause low CSF glucose levels.

Reference

Beaman MH: Acute community-acquired meningitis and encephalitis. Med J Aust 2002;176:389. [PMID: 12041637]

Nosocomial Pneumonia

- ■ Essentials of Diagnosis
  - Common nosocomial infection, with mortality rate up to 70%
  - Aspiration of oropharyngeal material most common route of acquisition; oropharynx often colonized with gram-negative, hospital-acquired organisms; 20–40% polymicrobial
  - Risk factors: neurologic impairment, mechanical ventilation, witnessed aspiration, lung and heart disease, supine position, older age, nasogastric tube
  - Less commonly, inhalation and nosocomial acquisition of tuberculosis, legionellosis, influenza, aspergillosis
  - Nosocomial bacteremia with *Staphylococcus aureus* and *Candida* spp can lead to hematogenous pneumonia

- ■ Differential Diagnosis
  - Acute respiratory distress syndrome
  - Pulmonary emboli
  - Cardiogenic pulmonary edema
  - Malignancy (primary lung or metastatic disease)
  - Atelectasis

- ■ Treatment
  - Antibiotic therapy targeting local nosocomial flora
  - Sputum Gram stain, culture may guide therapy; quantitative endotracheal aspirate (sensitivity 52–100%), bronchoalveolar lavage (80–100%), protected brush specimen (65–100%) more useful
  - Supportive care with frequent suctioning of respiratory secretion, postural drainage and, in some patients, bronchoscopy for drainage
  - Use preventive measures such as semirecumbent position (elevate head of bed), avoid long-term nasal intubation, use frequent supraglottic suctioning

- ■ Pearl
  Consider nosocomial pulmonary aspergillosis in neutropenic patients.

Reference
Johanson WG: Nosocomial pneumonia. Intens Care Med 2003;29:23. [PMID: 12528018]

Peritonitis

- **Essentials of Diagnosis**
  - Spontaneous bacterial peritonitis (SBP); or secondary peritonitis from perforation of abdominal viscus
  - SBP defined as ascitic fluid with >250 neutrophils/mm^3 or positive Gram stain (rarely) or culture of ascitic fluid; 50% with fever, abdominal tenderness; 30% asymptomatic
  - SBP seen in 8–27% of patients with cirrhosis and ascites; likely due to translocation of bacteria across gut lumen; *E coli* most common, then *K pneumoniae*, streptococci, enterococci, anaerobes; mortality up to 50%
  - Secondary peritonitis patients have severe abdominal pain, nausea, vomiting, fever, abdominal tenderness, hypotension; secondary to perforation of viscus; ascitic fluid with leukocytosis, Gram stain and cultures polymicrobial; abdominal radiographs or CT scan may show free intraperitoneal air

- **Differential Diagnosis**
  - Appendicitis, intra-abdominal abscess
  - Sickle cell crisis
  - Diabetic ketoacidosis
  - Porphyria
  - Familial Mediterranean fever
  - Lead poisoning
  - Uremia
  - Systemic lupus erythematosus with serositis

- **Treatment**
  - SBP, use third-generation cephalosporin
  - Secondary peritonitis requires evaluation and surgical management for perforated viscus; antibiotic coverage must include anaerobes and enteric gram-negative bacilli

- **Pearl**

Suspect secondary peritonitis if more than one microorganism on Gram stain or culture of ascitic fluid.

Reference

Malangoni MA: Current concepts in peritonitis. Curr Gastroenterol Rep 2003;5:295. [PMID: 12864959]

Pneumocystis jiroveci Pneumonia (PCP)

■ Essentials of Diagnosis

- Nonproductive cough, fever, progressive dyspnea; chest radiograph with interstitial infiltrates, often bilateral
- Arterial hypoxemia, sometimes out of proportion to chest radiographic findings
- Diagnosis confirmed by Giemsa or methenamine silver stain or immunofluorescent antibody stain of sputum or bronchoalveolar lavage
- Commonly seen in patients with advanced HIV infection, low CD_4 cell count, and those not receiving Pneumocystis prophylaxis
- Prolonged administration of corticosteroids associated with increased risk in HIV-negative hosts

■ Differential Diagnosis

- Bacterial, viral, or fungal pneumonia
- Tuberculosis
- Congestive heart failure
- Acute respiratory distress syndrome
- Pulmonary emboli

■ Treatment

- High-dose trimethoprim-sulfamethoxazole (15 mg/kg/day of trimethoprim component)
- Alternatives: atovaquone, clindamycin plus primaquine, dapsone plus trimethoprim, pentamidine
- Oxygen or mechanical ventilation, if indicated, for respiratory failure
- Adjunctive therapy with corticosteroids if $P(A-a)O_2$ >35 mm Hg or PO_2 ≤ 70 mm Hg
- For HIV-infected patients, secondary prophylaxis against Pneumocystis until CD4 count consistently >200 cells/mm^3 with antiretroviral therapy

■ Pearl

A patient with suspected PCP who has a normal serum LDH should be evaluated for an alternative diagnosis.

Reference

Morris A: Improved survival with highly active antiretroviral therapy in HIV-infected patients with severe Pneumocystis carinii pneumonia. AIDS 2003;17:73. [PMID: 12478071]

Prevention of Nosocomial Infection

- **Essential Concepts**
  - Infection acquired in hospital (not present or incubating at the time of admission); onset at least 2–4 days after hospitalization depending on site and pathogen identified
  - Manifestations specific for site and source
  - Occurs in 5–35% of ICU patients; most common urinary tract infection, pneumonia, surgical site infection, bloodstream
  - Sources: bacterial flora colonizing patients, with pathogens increasingly resistant to antibiotics, and patient's endogenous flora

- **Essentials of Management**
  - Prevent cross-contamination using universal precautions (hand washing; gloves, masks, gowns when necessary; special care with patient soiled linen and removed devices); appropriate isolation of patients with easily transmissible pathogens (*C difficile*, *M tuberculosis*) or highly resistant pathogens (methicillin-resistant *S aureus*, vancomycin-resistant enterococcus)
  - Appropriate use of antimicrobial agents to limit selection of resistant pathogens
  - Ventilator-associated pneumonia: use semirecumbent rather than supine positioning, sucralfate rather than antacid therapy for prevention of stress gastritis (controversial), continuous subglottic aspiration, noninvasive ventilation when possible
  - Nosocomial sinusitis: limit duration of nasogastric or nasolaryngeal tubes; oral hygiene
  - Bloodstream infection: use careful sterile technique in insertion and handling of devices; use "tunneled" catheters for long-term intravenous use; minimize use of femoral venous catheters; consider use of antimicrobial impregnated catheters in selected patients
  - Urinary tract infection: use indwelling urinary catheter only when necessary; reassess need daily, discontinue if possible
  - Surgical site infections: stress optimal sterile surgical techniques; antimicrobial prophylaxis when and only if appropriate

- **Pearl**

Hand washing is the single most effective method to avoid nosocomial transmission of pathogens.

Reference

Eggimann P: Infection control in the ICU. Chest 2001;120:2059. [PMID: 11742943]

Pulmonary Infections in HIV-Infected Patients

- **Essentials of Diagnosis**
  - Pneumococcal or other bacterial pneumonia: abrupt onset of productive cough, fever, pleuritic chest pain (pneumococcal or other bacterial pneumonia)
  - Tuberculous or fungal pneumonia (including *Pneumocystis jiroveci*): more gradual onset of fever, less purulent sputum, cough, weight loss
  - Pneumocystis pneumonia: gradual onset of dyspnea, fever, no or very minimal sputum
  - Chest radiographic findings vary from focal infiltrates to diffuse interstitial markings
  - Diagnosis by sputum smear and culture (pneumococcus, TB), bronchoscopic sampling (PCP), serologies (coccidioides, histoplasma, cryptococcal pneumonia)
  - Immune-suppression (CD_4 cell count) determines likelihoods; CD_4 count >200/mm^3 (*S pneumoniae, M tuberculosis, S aureus*, influenza); <200/mm^3 (*Pneumocystis jiroveci* (PCP), *C neoformans, M tuberculosis*; <50/mm^3 (*Pneumocystis jiroveci*, histoplasmosis, *P aeruginosa*, CMV (coinfection with PCP), *M avium* complex)
  - *M tuberculosis* and *S pneumoniae* at increased incidence across all CD_4 strata

- **Differential Diagnosis**
  - Tumors (primary lung carcinoma, Kaposi sarcoma, lymphoma)
  - Interstitial lung disease
  - Acute respiratory distress syndrome; congestive heart failure; pulmonary emboli

- **Treatment**
  - Evaluate and manage respiratory failure
  - Respiratory isolation of patient if tuberculosis suspected
  - Empiric antimicrobial therapy against likely organism, guided by clinical presentation and CD_4 count
  - Diagnostic thoracentesis if pleural effusion present

- **Pearl**

In presence of either pleural effusion or purulent sputum production, consider diagnoses other than Pneumocystis pneumonia.

Reference

Wolff AJ: HIV-related pulmonary infections: a review of the recent literature. Curr Opin Pulm Med 2003;9:210. [PMID: 12682566]

Sepsis

- **Essentials of Diagnosis**
  - Defined as infection with accompanying systemic inflammatory response syndrome (SIRS), with two or more of following: temperature >38°C or <36°C; heart rate >90/minute; respiratory rate >20/minute; white blood cell count >12,000/μL or <4000/μL or >10% bands
  - Clinical features range from sepsis (SIRS plus culture-documented infection) to severe sepsis (sepsis with organ dysfunction or hypotension) to septic shock (sepsis with hypotension and hypoperfusion)
  - Any microorganism can cause sepsis; bacteria most commonly implicated; blood cultures positive in only 40%
  - Immune suppression or uncontrolled immune response may contribute to sepsis syndrome
  - Leading cause of death in ICU patients in the United States

- **Differential Diagnosis**
  - Multiple trauma
  - Severe hemorrhagic or necrotizing pancreatitis
  - Severe burns
  - Acute myocardial infarction
  - Pulmonary emboli
  - Metabolic and hematologic derangements

- **Treatment**
  - Early recognition of sepsis crucial for successful treatment
  - Supportive care with oxygen and ventilatory support, intravenous fluid administration, vasopressor agents to increase oxygen delivery
  - Antibiotic therapy guided towards clinically and epidemiologically suspected pathogens
  - Surgical drainage of abscesses or necrotic tissue
  - Intensive insulin therapy for hyperglycemia
  - Consider adjunctive therapy with recombinant human activated protein C in selected patients (severe sepsis without active risk of bleeding); other adjunctive therapies targeting the immune response under investigation.

- **Pearl**

Mortality approaches 100% in septic patients with shock or failure of ≤3 organ systems.

Reference

Hotchkiss RS: The pathophysiology and treatment of sepsis. NEJM 2003;348:138. [PMID: 12519925]

Surgical Site Infection (SSI)

- **Essentials of Diagnosis**
  - Infection of surgical incision site(s), both superficial and deep
  - Endogenous or hospital-acquired flora involved; usually occurs within 4–8 days of surgery, if caused by staphylococci and gram-negative organisms; earlier infection (<48 hours) caused by clostridia and beta-hemolytic streptococci
  - Risk factors include host (extremes of age, poor nutritional status, diabetes, smoking, obesity, coexisting remote infection, bacterial colonization, altered immune response, prolonged preoperative hospital stay); operative factors (hygiene and antiseptic procedures, prophylactic antibiotics); postoperative factors (incision care)

- **Differential Diagnosis**
  - Other causes of postoperative fever (eg, atelectasis, thrombophlebitis, aspiration and drug reaction)
  - Inadequate postoperative pain control

- **Treatment**
  - Exploration of surgical wound or site of suspected infection; fluid draining from wound should have Gram stain and culture
  - Debridement of necrotic tissue and/or removal of foreign body
  - Antibiotic therapy targeting nosocomial gram positive as well as gram negative organisms

- **Pearl**

Antimicrobial prophylaxis indicated in surgery involving opening hollow viscus, placement of foreign bodies, or when potential SSI poses catastrophic risk; should consist of 1–2 doses of antibiotics only, administered pre- and sometimes postoperatively, to decrease intraoperative organism burden.

Reference

Mangram AJ: Guideline for prevention of surgical site infection 1999. Hospital Infection Control Practices Advisory Committee. Infect Control Hosp Epidemiol 1999;20:250. [PMID: 10219875]

Tetanus

- **Essentials of Diagnosis**
  - Neurologic disorder caused by neurotoxin produced by *Clostridium tetani*; toxin binds to presynaptic inhibitory neurons causing uncontrolled motor neuron activity
  - Presentations: (1) neonatal tetanus; and (2) generalized; (3) local; or (4) cephalic tetanus in adults; local and cephalic tetanus can progress to generalized
  - Trismus ("lockjaw") most common; advanced tetanus with generalized spasms, opisthotonos, abdominal rigidity, spastic facial expression ("risus sardonicus"); involvement of respiratory muscles leads to hypoventilation; autonomic nervous system disturbances common (sweating, tachycardia, arrhythmias, fluctuating blood pressure); fever notably absent, except in patients with seizures
  - 1 to 54 days following wound contaminated with *C tetani* spores; crush, frostbite wounds with higher risk; wound cultures frequently negative for *C tetani*
  - Lack of *C tetani* antibody (no immunization) supports diagnosis
  - *C tetani* spores survive years in dust, soil, areas contaminated by human or animal excreta; common in developing countries; rare in the U.S. (50 cases per year); entirely preventable by tetanus vaccination

- **Differential Diagnosis**
  - Strychnine poisoning, phenothiazine overdose
  - Mandibular or other lesions causing jaw lock
  - Meningoencephalitis, opioid withdrawal, diphtheria, mumps, rabies

- **Treatment**
  - Tetanus immune globulin
  - Debridement of wound; penicillin G (kills active bacteria; spores not affected by antibiotics)
  - Supportive care with tracheostomy, mechanical ventilation, benzodiazepines, nutritional support, therapy of seizures and cardiac arrhythmias
  - Active immunization during convalescent phase

- **Pearl**

Binding of toxin is irreversible; rapid administration of antitoxin crucial to prevent progression and likelihood of death.

Reference

Farrar JJ et al: Tetanus. J Neurol Neurosurg Psychiatry 2000;69:292–301. [PMID: 10945801]

Toxic Shock Syndrome

- **Essentials of Diagnosis**
  - Multisystem illness characterized by rapid onset of fever, vomiting, watery diarrhea, pharyngitis, profound myalgias with accompanying hypotension
  - Diffuse blanching truncal erythema early, accentuated in axillary and inguinal folds, spreading to extremities
  - Desquamation of skin, palms and soles occurs in second or third week
  - Multiorgan system involvement, with acute renal failure, ARDS, refractory shock, ventricular arrhythmias, and DIC may occur
  - Highest incidence in menstruating women, persons with localized or postsurgical staphylococcal infection, and women using diaphragm or contraceptive sponge

- **Differential Diagnosis**
  - Scarlet fever/Streptococcal toxic-shock-like disease
  - Kawasaki's disease
  - Rocky Mountain spotted fever
  - Drug eruptions/Stevens-Johnson syndrome
  - Measles
  - Leptospirosis
  - Sepsis syndrome with multiorgan system failure

- **Treatment**
  - Immediate removal of tampon, contraceptive device, or surgical packing
  - Surgical drainage, irrigation of focal abscess
  - Supportive care, with fluid resuscitation and management of organ system failure
  - Antistaphylococcal antibiotic, though effect on outcome unclear

- **Pearl**

Intense hyperemia of conjunctival, oropharyngeal, and vaginal surfaces are frequent findings in toxic shock syndrome.

Reference

Provost TT, Flynn JA (editors): *Cutaneous Medicine: Cutaneous Manifestations of Systemic Disease.* BC Decker, 2001.

Urosepsis

- **Essentials of Diagnosis**
  - Urinary tract infection with secondary sepsis; ascending route of infection most common
  - Vesiculoureteral reflux and renal transplant (short ureter with high risk of reflux) predispose to pyelonephritis; women higher risk for cystitis secondary to short urethra
  - *E coli* most common pathogen but multidrug-resistant gram-negative rods, candida, coagulase negative staphylococci may cause nosocomial urosepsis
  - Complications: intrarenal or perinephric abscess, obstruction, and infected renal stones; emphysematous pyelonephritis rare complication of elderly women with diabetes mellitus, chronic urinary tract infection, underlying renal vascular disease; organism typically *E coli*

- **Differential Diagnosis**
  - Sepsis from other sources
  - Simple acute pyelonephritis or cystitis

- **Treatment**
  - Systemic antibiotics targeting most likely pathogen (urine Gram stain may guide empiric therapy)
  - If negative urine Gram stain, empiric therapy with aminoglycoside, extended-spectrum penicillin, third-generation cephalosporin, or fluoroquinolone
  - Obtain imaging studies (ultrasound examination, computed tomography, or CT urogram) to evaluate possible complications
  - Emphysematous pyelonephritis requires immediate nephrectomy

- **Pearl**

In uroseptic patient, urine culture growing S aureus should prompt work up for S aureus bacteremia (eg, infective endocarditis).

Reference

Paradisi F: Urosepsis in the critical care unit. Crit Care Clin 1998;14:165. [PMID: 9561812]

11

Gastrointestinal Disease

| Acalculous Cholecystitis |

- **Essentials of Diagnosis**
  - Acute inflammation and necrosis of gallbladder with unexplained fever, leukocytosis, vague abdominal or right upper quadrant pain; often insidious onset in susceptible patient
  - Right upper quadrant abdominal tenderness highly variable; mass in 20%; jaundice, positive Murphy sign
  - Leukocytosis, elevated bilirubin, alkaline phosphatase, aminotransferases
  - Thickening of gallbladder wall, pericholecystic fluid, absence of gallstones on abdominal ultrasound; positive ultrasonographic Murphy sign; sometimes may fail to visualize gallbladder
  - Severe cases with emphysematous cholecystitis, perforation with abscess formation
  - Predisposing conditions: critical illness, especially with hypotension, sepsis, postoperative, immunosuppression, total parenteral nutrition, diabetes, biliary surgery; may have no predisposing factors
  - Caused by combination of bile stasis, ischemia, local inflammation; part of multiorgan failure in ICU patients

- **Differential Diagnosis**
  - Calculous cholecystitis
  - Acute pancreatitis
  - Pyogenic hepatic, subphrenic, or intra-abdominal abscess
  - Ascending cholangitis

- **Treatment**
  - Antibiotics directed against enteric pathogens and anaerobes (ampicillin, aminoglycoside, metronidazole)
  - Cholecystectomy (open or laparoscopic); laparoscopic preferred in critically ill patients
  - Drain abscesses

- **Pearl**

In patients too ill to undergo surgery, temporizing strategies with antibiotics and percutaneous drainage until more stable for cholecystectomy may be useful.

Reference

McChesney JA et al: Acute acalculous cholecystitis associated with systemic sepsis and visceral arterial hypoperfusion: a case series and review of pathophysiology. Dig Dis Sci 2003;48:1960. [PMID: 14627341]

Adynamic (Paralytic) Ileus

- **Essentials of Diagnosis**
  - Mild to moderate continuous abdominal pain, vomiting, obstipation
  - Massive abdominal distention with localized tenderness common; decreased or absent bowel sounds
  - Hemoconcentration; volume and electrolyte depletion with prolonged vomiting, sequestration into distended bowel loops
  - Leukocytosis and elevated amylase can be present
  - Radiographs demonstrate gas-filled loops of bowel and multiple air-fluid levels; air may be evident in rectum
  - Barium swallow with small bowel follow-through or contrast enema will differentiate ileus from mechanical obstruction
  - Associated with neurogenic or muscular impairment of small- or large-bowel function
  - Precipitating factors: recent abdominal surgery, ruptured viscus, peritonitis, pancreatitis, medications, anoxic injury, spinal cord trauma, uremia, diabetic coma, hypokalemia

- **Differential Diagnosis**
  - Idiopathic small-bowel pseudoobstruction
  - Colonic pseudoobstruction (Ogilvie syndrome)
  - Small- or large-bowel mechanical obstruction

- **Treatment**
  - Identify and treat precipitating event or remove causative agent; decrease or avoid opioids
  - Restrict oral intake
  - Replete fluids and electrolytes with isotonic fluids
  - Nasogastric suction useful for symptomatic relief but probably does not improve clinical outcome
  - Postoperative ileus: NSAIDs help reduce opioid use and may decrease bowel inflammation
  - Prokinetic agents including erythromycin or metoclopramide
  - After failure of conservative therapy, a trial of neostigmine may be beneficial for Ogilvie syndrome
  - Colonoscopy if colonic dilation present
  - Surgery rarely needed

- **Pearl**

Recent abdominal surgery is the most common cause of adynamic ileus in the ICU; function returns to the small bowel generally within 24 hours but may take several days to return to normal motility in the colon.

Reference

Luckey A et al: Mechanism and treatment of postoperative ileus. Arch Surg 2003;138:206. [PMID: 12578422]

Ascites

- **Essentials of Diagnosis**
  - Increasing abdominal girth and pressure, anorexia, early satiety, nausea, dyspnea
  - Shifting dullness, fluid wave, bulging flanks
  - If due to liver disease: jaundice, spider angiomas, caput medusa, palmar erythema, testicular atrophy, gynecomastia
  - Ascitic fluid assessment: cell count and differential, albumin, protein, Gram stain plus culture; amylase, cytology, glucose, LDH, triglycerides
  - Calculate serum-ascites albumin gradient (SAAG): portal hypertension (>1.1 g/dL) or nonportal hypertensive causes (<1.1 g/dL)
  - Spontaneous bacterial peritonitis (SBP) frequent complication; ascitic fluid with >250 neutrophils/μL diagnostic
  - Ultrasound and CT scan: useful in localizing small volume ascites, identifying vascular thrombosis, determining etiology
  - Grossly bloody ascites: repeat paracentesis in another location; if hemoperitoneum confirmed, emergent CT scan and surgical consult

- **Differential Diagnosis**
  - Portal Hypertension (High SAAG): cirrhosis, cardiac failure, portal or hepatic venoocclusive disease, fatty liver of pregnancy
  - Nonportal Hypertensive Ascites (Low SAAG): malignancy, intraperitoneal infection, nephrotic syndrome, pancreatitis

- **Treatment**
  - Sodium and fluid restriction for mild ascites
  - Spironolactone and loop diuretics for moderate ascites
  - Monitor weight, electrolytes, creatinine during diuresis
  - Paracentesis for tense refractory ascites; consider salt-poor albumin infusions during large volume paracentesis
  - Transjugular intrahepatic portosystemic shunt (TIPS) for intractable ascites; other options include surgical peritoneovenous shunting, liver transplantation
  - Treat SBP with antibiotics, albumin infusion; consider prophylactic antibiotics for prior SBP, upper GI hemorrhage, low protein ascites

- **Pearl**

Over 50% of patients with cirrhosis will develop ascites. Once ascites develops, the median survival is only 1 year.

Reference

Moore KP et al: The management of ascites in cirrhosis. Hepatology 2003;38:258. [PMID: 12830009]

Boerhaave Syndrome

■ Essentials of Diagnosis

- Esophageal perforation leading to suppurative mediastinitis
- History of excessive or rapid alcohol or food ingestion
- Vomiting or retching followed by severe, typically left sided chest pain; exacerbated by respiration and swallowing
- Dyspnea can be prominent feature
- Fever, hypotension, tachycardia, tachypnea
- Subcutaneous emphysema, Hamman crunch
- Leukocytosis and elevated serum amylase
- Radiographic findings: pneumomediastinum, pneumopericardium, pneumothorax, pleural effusion, subcutaneous emphysema
- Esophagogram with water-soluble contrast material has 75% sensitivity; consider repeating if negative
- CT scan of chest helpful if esophagogram negative
- Pleural fluid demonstrates low pH and high amylase; may detect food particles

■ Differential Diagnosis

- Aortic dissection
- Myocardial infarction
- Perforated peptic ulcer
- Iatrogenic esophageal rupture
- Pulmonary embolism
- Spontaneous pneumothorax
- Pancreatitis

■ Treatment

- Immediate broad-spectrum antibiotics
- Supportive measures including aggressive hydration with isotonic crystalloid
- Restrict all oral intake
- Total parenteral nutrition to support nutritional status
- Nasogastric intubation with suctioning
- Aggressive and early surgical treatment
- Rare patients may recover with conservative therapy and pleural drainage only

■ Pearl

Factors predicting a poor outcome in Boerhaave syndrome include spontaneous perforation and a greater than 24 hour delay in diagnosis and initiation of treatment.

Reference

Janjua KJ: Boerhaave's syndrome. Postgrad Med J 1997;73:265. [PMID: 9196697]

Cholangitis, Acute

- **Essentials of Diagnosis**
  - Fever, jaundice, abdominal pain in 50–75%; fewer symptoms in elderly, patients receiving corticosteroids
  - Right upper quadrant tenderness, jaundice, hypotension, manifestations of sepsis
  - Leukocytosis; elevated bilirubin, alkaline phosphatase, amylase
  - Common bile duct dilatation, stone, stricture seen on abdominal ultrasonography; MR cholangiopancreatography also useful
  - Caused by ascending bacteria into biliary tract; almost always associated with obstruction from gallstones, strictures, malignancy, after biliary procedures (ERCP)

- **Differential Diagnosis**
  - Liver abscess
  - Acute pancreatitis
  - Acute cholecystitis
  - Biliary leaks

- **Treatment**
  - Support patient with fluids and vasopressors if hypotensive
  - Antibiotics for gram-negative enteric bacteria (*E coli*, *K pneumoniae*), enterococcus; often ampicillin, aminoglycoside; avoid fluoroquinolones, third-generation cephalosporins alone; treatment for anaerobic bacteria usually unnecessary
  - Consider biliary drainage if unresponsive to antibiotics and persistent pain, hypotension, fever, altered sensorium using ERCP, percutaneous drainage, or open surgical procedure
  - ERCP useful for sphincterotomy, drainage, stent placement
  - All patients should have correction of obstruction 72 hours after resolution of fever; overall outcome depends on mechanism of obstruction (benign or malignant)

- **Pearl**

Abnormal sensorium in patients with acute cholangitis has been associated with poorer outcome.

Reference

Sugiyama M et al: Treatment of acute cholangitis due to choledocholithiasis in elderly and younger patients. Arch Surg 1997;132:1129. [PMID: 9336514]

Diarrhea

- **Essentials of Diagnosis**
  - Increase in fluidity, frequency, or quantity (>200 g/day) of stool, any loose stool, or >500 mL watery stool per day for two days
  - Stool studies: fecal leukocytes, *C difficile* toxin, stool electrolytes to determine stool osmolar gap, ova and parasites
  - Consider flexible sigmoidoscopy if ischemic colitis or inflammatory bowel disease suspected
  - Etiologies: medications (antacids, antibiotics, metoclopramide), enteral feedings, infections, cholestatic syndromes (hepatitis, bile duct obstruction, steatorrhea), malabsorption (short-bowel syndrome, afferent loop syndrome), diabetic neuropathy, hyperthyroidism, immunodeficiency, inflammatory colitis
  - Complications: volume depletion, electrolyte losses, skin breakdown with secondary infection.

- **Differential Diagnosis**
  - Celiac disease
  - Pancreatic insufficiency
  - *C difficile* colitis
  - Ischemic colitis
  - Lactase deficiency
  - Hyperthyroidism
  - Drug-related diarrhea

- **Treatment**
  - Replete fluid and electrolyte losses
  - Discontinue possible causative agents and medications
  - Use antidiarrheal agents with great caution
  - Metronidazole or vancomycin for suspected or confirmed *C difficile* colitis; enteric precautions to prevent spread to other patients
  - Enteral feeding associated diarrhea: discontinuation only proven effective therapy; other options include changing to peptide-based formula, adding fiber, or changing rate, fat content, osmolality, or temperature of feeding solution
  - Consider parenteral nutrition if unable to tolerate enteral feedings
  - Disimpaction if related to constipation and fecal impaction
  - Specific treatment directed once etiology determined

- **Pearl**

C difficile colitis in the ICU can be acquired from environmental exposures, person-to-person contacts, and hand carriage from health care providers.

Reference

Ringel AF et al: Diarrhea in the intensive care patient. Crit Care Clin 1995;11:465. [PMID: 7788541]

Gastric or Esophageal Variceal Bleeding

- **Essentials of Diagnosis**
  - History of chronic liver disease or previous variceal bleed; varices are dilated collateral veins caused by elevated portal venous pressure; most commonly seen in cirrhosis
  - Acute onset of painless large volume hematemesis
  - Melena or hematochezia may be present
  - Orthostatic hypotension, tachycardia
  - Stigmata of chronic liver disease: jaundice, ascites, palmar erythema, splenomegaly, telangiectasias, gonadal atrophy
  - Confusion related to hypotension or encephalopathy
  - Anemia may not be present with acute bleeding
  - Chronic hepatic dysfunction common: hyperbilirubinemia, hypoalbuminemia, elevated serum aminotransferases and alkaline phosphatase, prolonged coagulation times, thrombocytopenia
  - Nasogastric aspiration may demonstrate blood or "coffee grounds"
  - Esophagogastroduodenoscopy (EGD) demonstrates esophagogastric varices

- **Differential Diagnosis**
  - Gastritis
  - Mallory-Weiss tear
  - Peptic ulcer disease
  - Malignancy

- **Treatment**
  - Stabilize hemodynamics: adequate intravenous access; infuse isotonic crystalloid; transfuse blood products as necessary
  - Support and protect airway
  - Serial assessment of vital signs, hemoglobin, platelets, coagulation panel
  - Early administration of octreotide or terlipressin
  - Intravenous or oral proton pump inhibitors
  - EGD for confirmation and therapeutic intervention: sclerotherapy, band ligation
  - Consider use of balloon tamponade device or proceed to transjugular intrahepatic portosystemic shunt (TIPS) in uncontrolled variceal bleeding
  - Surgery reserved when above measures fail
  - Consider empiric antibiotics for spontaneous bacterial peritonitis

- **Pearl**

If isolated gastric varices are identified on endoscopy, suspect splenic vein thrombosis.

Reference

Sharara AI et al: Gastroesophageal variceal hemorrhage. N Engl J Med 2001;345:669. [PMID: 11547722]

Gastritis

- **Essentials of Diagnosis**
    - Mild epigastric tenderness, fecal occult blood, melena
    - May be asymptomatic
    - Decreasing hemoglobin may be only finding with acute gastritis
    - Iron deficiency anemia seen with chronic gastritis
    - Esophagogastroduodenoscopy (EGD) reveals erythema and erosions; biopsy diagnostic
    - Etiologies: critical illness, sepsis, or burns which may cause hypoperfusion to gastric mucosa; pharmacologic agents (NSAIDs); *H pylori* infection; alcohol use; atrophic gastropathy; previous surgery; prolonged mechanical ventilation

- **Differential Diagnosis**
    - Peptic ulcer disease
    - Esophagitis
    - Malignancy

- **Treatment**
    - Supportive measures: ensure adequate intravenous access; infuse isotonic crystalloid; transfuse blood if anemic, plasma to correct coagulopathy, platelets if thrombocytopenic
    - Intravenous or oral acid suppressive agents: histamine type-2 antagonists, proton pump inhibitors
    - Treat underlying cause of hypoperfusion and shock
    - Avoid and remove offending agents
    - EGD can identify lesions and treat with different measures to obtain hemostasis
    - Eradicate *H pylori* if suspected or confirmed during EGD
    - Vasopressin infusion, selective angiography, or surgery rarely indicated

- **Pearl**

Stress gastritis, although common in ICU setting, is rarely a life-threatening event.

Reference

Wu JC et al: Ulcers and gastritis. Endoscopy 2002;34:104. [PMID: 11822005]

Hepatic Failure, Acute

- **Essentials of Diagnosis**
  - Rapid onset of severe impairment of liver function
  - Hepatic encephalopathy predominant: asterixis, slowing of mentation, sleep disruption, confusion, coma
  - Malaise, fatigue, anorexia
  - Hypotension, tachycardia, occasionally fever
  - Jaundice, hepatomegaly, right upper quadrant tenderness
  - Dramatic elevations of serum aminotransferases and bilirubin; hypoalbuminemia, hypoglycemia
  - Leukocytosis, thrombocytopenia, coagulopathy
  - Progression to multiorgan system failure, including hepatorenal syndrome
  - Poor prognostic signs: age <10 or >40, jaundice >7 days before onset of encephalopathy, serum bilirubin >17.5, coma, respiratory failure, coagulopathy, hepatitis C, halothane exposure, idiosyncratic drug reaction

- **Differential Diagnosis**
  - Acute viral hepatitis
  - Drugs/toxins
  - Acute fatty liver of pregnancy
  - Ischemia/hypoperfusion
  - Acute choledocholithiasis
  - Acute Wilson disease

- **Treatment**
  - Stabilize and protect airway; intubate to facilitate correction of acidosis, prevent aspiration
  - Hemodynamic support: adequate intravenous access; infuse isotonic crystalloid; transfuse red blood cells if significantly anemic; correct coagulopathy if actively bleeding or planning invasive procedure; vasopressors
  - Add dextrose to intravenous fluids to avoid hypoglycemia
  - Manage encephalopathy and cerebral edema: may need direct intracranial pressure monitoring; elevate head of bed to 20–30°; hyperventilate; minimize patient stimulation; consider mannitol
  - Administer N-acetylcysteine until acetaminophen toxicity excluded
  - Consider liver transplantation early in treatment course

- **Pearl**

Acute hepatic failure may alter the pharmacokinetics of commonly used ICU medications metabolized by the liver.

Reference

Marrero J et al: Advances in critical care hepatology. Am J Respir Crit Care Med 2003;168:1421. [PMID: 14668256]

Large-Bowel Obstruction

- ■ Essentials of Diagnosis
  - • Symptoms vary with location and degree of obstruction
  - • Constipation or obstipation
  - • Cramping pain referred to hypogastrium
  - • Continuous pain suggestive of intestinal ischemia
  - • Vomiting late finding; may not occur if ileocecal valve does not allow reflux
  - • High-pitched metallic tinkling, rushes, gurgles may be auscultated; abdominal distention; peristaltic waves may be seen
  - • Radiographs demonstrate large dilated loops of large bowel; absence of rectal gas
  - • Barium enema confirms diagnosis and may be therapeutic
  - • Colonoscopy or sigmoidoscopy can confirm diagnosis and may be therapeutic; can be complicated by perforation
  - • Etiologies: malignancy, volvulus, diverticular disease, inflammatory bowel disease, fecal impaction, strictures, adhesions, benign tumors
  - • Complications: progressive increase in intraluminal pressure leading to impaired circulation and subsequent gangrene and perforation

- ■ Differential Diagnosis
  - • Small-bowel obstruction
  - • Colonic pseudoobstruction
  - • Volvulus
  - • Ischemic enteritis
  - • Adynamic ileus

- ■ Treatment
  - • Replete fluids and electrolytes with isotonic fluids
  - • Barium enema, colonoscopy, or sigmoidoscopy may decompress and correct obstruction
  - • Mechanical obstruction generally requires surgery; other indications for surgery: perforation, ischemia, unchanged or worsening distention after 12–24 hours of conservative management
  - • Some descending colonic lesions may respond to endoscopic techniques including stent placement
  - • Broad spectrum antibiotics should be administered promptly if strangulation or perforation suspected

- ■ Pearl

In the presence of large-bowel obstruction, suspect carcinoma if rectal examination reveals occult blood, while fresh blood is more characteristic of diverticular disease.

Reference

Lopez-Kostner F et al: Management and causes of acute large-bowel obstruction. Surg Clin North Am 1997;77:1265. [PMID: 9431339]

Lower Gastrointestinal Bleeding, Acute

- **Essentials of Diagnosis**
  - Hematochezia and bright red blood per rectum with source below ligament of Treitz
  - Symptoms depend on amount and acuity of blood loss, underlying comorbid diseases: asymptomatic, lightheadedness, syncope, dyspnea, angina; abdominal pain and anorectal complaints may be present
  - Decreased caliber stools seen in colon cancer
  - Physical findings variable: normal; orthostatic hypotension; anorectal mass; multiple telangiectasias
  - Acute bleeding initially with normal blood cell count; chronic bleeding leads to iron deficient microcytic anemia
  - Colonoscopy diagnostic in up to 80% of patients; distal sources seen with sigmoidoscopy
  - Consider nuclear medicine scan or angiography if adequate preparation not possible
  - Bleeding stops spontaneously in 85% of cases

- **Differential Diagnosis**
  - Massive upper gastrointestinal hemorrhage
  - Arteriovenous malformations, angiodysplasia
  - Diverticulosis
  - Hemorrhoids
  - Malignancy
  - Inflammatory bowel disease

- **Treatment**
  - Stabilize hemodynamics: adequate intravenous access; infuse isotonic crystalloid; transfuse blood products
  - Serial assessment of vital signs, hemoglobin, platelets, coagulation panel
  - Nasogastric lavage to evaluate for upper gastrointestinal source when large amounts maroon colored stool present
  - Colonoscopy: identify culprit lesion, provide therapeutic intervention with electrocoagulation, sclerotherapy, resection
  - Angiodysplasia can be managed if identified during angiography with embolization or injection techniques
  - Surgery warranted for uncontrolled bleeding with unidentifiable cause; also indicated in recurrent diverticular disease, persistent bleeding from angiodysplasia

- **Pearl**

Gastrointestinal bleeding and calcific aortic stenosis (Heyde syndrome) has a high likelihood of angiodysplasia and has been reported to resolve with replacement of the diseased aortic valve.

Reference

Billingham RP: The conundrum of lower gastrointestinal bleeding. Surg Clin North Am 1997;77:241. [PMID: 9092113]

Pancreatic Insufficiency

- **Essentials of Diagnosis**
  - Steatorrhea with frequent bulky light-colored stools
  - Significant abdominal pain if associated with chronic pancreatitis
  - Increased symptoms with high fat content meals as fat absorption affected more than protein or carbohydrate
  - Increased fecal fat excretion; decreased serum cholesterol
  - Fecal elastase and chymotrypsin are decreased
  - Secretin or cholecystokinin test demonstrates pancreatic fluid bicarbonate of <80 mEq/L
  - Vitamin deficiency rare
  - Etiologies: pancreatic surgery, pancreatectomy, pancreatitis
  - Chronic pancreatitis may be identified by ERCP, MRCP, endoscopic ultrasound, or CT scan
  - Loss of >90% of pancreas exocrine function required before signs and symptoms of pancreatic insufficiency appear

- **Differential Diagnosis**
  - Lactase deficiency
  - Celiac disease/sprue
  - Chronic infectious diarrhea

- **Treatment**
  - Daily dietary intake of 3,000–6,000 kcal
  - Caloric supplementation with medium chain triglycerides
  - Pancreatic enzyme replacement; titrate dose based on dietary fat content
  - Dietary fat restriction to control diarrhea
  - Pain control

- **Pearl**

Because gastric acid can destroy oral lipase, administration of acid-suppressing agents may improve efficacy.

Reference

Petersen JM et al: Chronic pancreatitis and maldigestion. Semin Gastrointest Dis 2002;13:191. [PMID: 12462705]

Pancreatitis

■ Essentials of Diagnosis
- Severe epigastric or upper-abdominal pain radiating to back; associated with nausea, vomiting, anorexia
- Fever, volume depletion, shortness of breath may be present
- Hemodynamic and respiratory compromise in severe cases
- Epigastric and upper-quadrant tenderness, distention
- Ecchymosis of umbilicus (Cullen sign), flanks (Grey Turner sign) rare; suggest hemorrhagic pancreatitis when present
- Elevated amylase and lipase; leukocytosis
- Radiographs may demonstrate "sentinel loop"
- CT scan and ultrasound: confirms organ enlargement; helps identify possible causes and complications
- Etiologies: alcohol consumption, biliary disease (gallstones, ductal abnormalities, tumor), hypercalcemia, infections, hypertriglyceridemia, trauma, scorpion venom, medications
- Complications: hemorrhage, necrosis, extrapancreatic fluid collections, pseudocyst, abscess, ARDS

■ Differential Diagnosis
- Acute cholecystitis or cholangitis
- Mesenteric ischemia or infarction
- Penetrating or perforating ulcer
- Intestinal obstruction
- Inferior wall myocardial infarction

■ Treatment
- Volume resuscitation with isotonic crystalloid; consider albumin infusion if serum level <3.0 g/dL; central venous or pulmonary artery catheter may help guide fluid replacement
- Nasogastric suctioning for ileus or nausea
- Pain control and antiemetics
- Early nutritional support may expedite recovery
- Intubation and mechanical ventilation for hypoxemia and ARDS
- Broad-spectrum antibiotics for complicated pancreatitis
- Fluid collections may be drained via endoscopic procedures, percutaneous drainage, surgical decompression
- Surgery indicated for sterile necrotizing pancreatitis not responsive to medical therapy, infected necrotizing pancreatitis

■ Pearl
Acute pancreatitis patients with more than 6 of Ranson criteria have a mortality rate greater than 40% and a complication rate greater than 80%.

Reference

Mitchell RMS et al: Pancreatitis. Lancet 2003;361:1447. [PMID: 12727412]

Peptic Ulcer Disease (PUD)

- **Essentials of Diagnosis**
  - Epigastric pain that may (duodenal) or may not (gastric) be relieved by food or antacids; worsens 1 to 3 hours after meals
  - Vomiting with gastric ulcers; back pain with duodenal ulcers
  - Hematemesis, melena, hematochezia with acute PUD bleeding
  - Epigastric tenderness and positive fecal occult blood
  - Nasogastric tube aspiration demonstrates coffee ground material or blood
  - Esophagogastroduodenoscopy (EGD) diagnostic
  - ICU "stress ulcer" risk factors: ventilatory support, lack of enteral feeding, elderly, burns, head injury
  - Associated diseases: COPD, cystic fibrosis, alpha-1 antitrypsin deficiency, chronic renal failure, cirrhosis
  - Complications: perforation, penetration, obstruction

- **Differential Diagnosis**
  - Gastric erosions/gastritis
  - Esophagitis
  - Varices
  - Mallory-Weiss tear

- **Treatment**
  - Stabilize hemodynamics: adequate intravenous access; infuse isotonic crystalloid; transfuse blood products if necessary
  - Serial assessment of vital signs, hemoglobin, platelets, coagulation panel
  - Intravenous or oral proton pump inhibitors
  - Eradicate *H pylori* if present or suspected in cases of duodenal or prepyloric ulcers
  - Avoid all ulcerogenic medications and agents
  - Endoscopy to identify cause and achieve hemostasis: local injection of sclerosing or vasoconstricting agents, thermal probes, bipolar coagulation, application of hemostatic agents
  - Angiography with embolization and surgery reserved for uncontrolled bleeding

- **Pearl**

Risk of rebleeding based on endoscopic findings is least for clean based ulcer, increases if adherent clot or visible vessel, and most with active bleeding.

Reference

Shiotani A et al: Pathogenesis and therapy of gastric and duodenal ulcer disease. Med Clin N Am 2002;86:1447. [PMID 12510460]

Small-Bowel Obstruction

- **Essentials of Diagnosis**
  - Intermittent or colicky abdominal pain with crescendo-decrescendo pattern; insidious onset with progressive abdominal bloating, constipation, or obstipation
  - Vomiting progressively feculent as illness progresses
  - Poorly localized crampy pain at site of involvement; progresses distally over course of illness
  - Distended, tender abdomen; may have peritoneal signs and abdominal wall hernias
  - Peristaltic "rushes" are auscultatory hallmark; may occur along with gurgles and high-pitched tinkles
  - Volume and electrolyte depletion common
  - Radiographs demonstrate ladderlike pattern of dilated small bowel loops and air-fluid levels; "thumbprinting" and gas in bowel wall suggest bowel necrosis
  - CT should be considered if plain films nondiagnostic
  - Etiologies: adhesions from previous surgeries, malignancies, hernias through the abdominal wall, volvulus, foreign bodies, inflammatory bowel disease, radiation therapy
  - Complications: aspiration pneumonia, strangulation, perforation, peritonitis, bacteremia, sepsis

- **Differential Diagnosis**
  - Adynamic ileus
  - Large bowel obstruction
  - Mesenteric vascular occlusion
  - Ischemic enteritis
  - Inflammatory bowel disease
  - Pancreatitis
  - Cystic fibrosis
  - Appendicitis
  - Large bowel obstruction

- **Treatment**
  - Replete fluids and electrolytes with isotonic fluids
  - Nasogastric suctioning to decompress bowel
  - Serial abdominal examinations and radiographic studies
  - Broad-spectrum antibiotics if strangulation or perforation suspected
  - Consider surgical intervention early; indications include strangulation, failure of conservative therapy

- **Pearl**

A strangulated obstruction should be suspected in the presence of early appearance of shock, gross hematemesis, and marked leukocytosis.

Reference

Wilson MS et al: A review of the management of small bowel obstruction. Ann R Coll Surg Engl 1999;81:320. [PMID: 10645174]

Upper Gastrointestinal Bleeding

- **Essentials of Diagnosis**
  - Hematemesis, coffee ground emesis, melena with source above the ligament of Treitz; occasionally hematochezia
  - Symptoms depend on amount and acuity of blood loss: asymptomatic, lightheadedness, syncope, dyspnea, angina; early satiety seen in gastric cancer
  - Physical findings variable: none; orthostatic hypotension; stigmata of liver disease; mucosal pigmentation (Peutz-Jeghers syndrome); multiple telangiectasias (Osler-Weber-Rendu)
  - Acute bleeding initially with normal blood cell count; chronic leads to iron deficient microcytic anemia
  - Nasogastric lavage demonstrates coffee ground material, blood
  - Esophagogastroduodenoscopy (EGD) to determine bleeding source; nuclear medicine scan or angiography helpful if EGD nondiagnostic
  - Mortality risks: advanced age; signs of systemic shock; significant comorbidities; diagnosis of malignancy; endoscopic findings of large varices, active bleeding, or visible vessel

- **Differential Diagnosis**
  - Gastric erosions/gastritis
  - Varices
  - Mallory-Weiss tear
  - Peptic ulcer disease
  - Esophagitis
  - Malignancy

- **Treatment**
  - Support and protect airway
  - Stabilize hemodynamics: adequate intravenous access; infuse isotonic crystalloid; transfuse blood products as necessary
  - Serial assessment of vital signs, hemoglobin, platelets, coagulation panel
  - EGD can identify lesions and treat with sclerotherapy, band ligation, application of hemostatic agents
  - Intravenous or oral proton pump inhibitors
  - Consider early use of octreotide or terlipressin in suspected cases of variceal bleeding
  - Surgery reserved when above measures fail

- **Pearl**

Early endoscopy is indicated in patients over 60 years of age, history of chronic liver disease, bright red blood per rectum associated with hypotension, and bleeding requiring more than 4 units of blood in a 6-hour period.

Reference

Conrad SA: Acute upper gastrointestinal bleeding in critically ill patients: causes and treatment modalities. Crit Care Med 2002;30:S365. [PMID: 12072663]

12

Endocrine Problems

Adrenal Insufficiency

- **Essentials of Diagnosis**
  - Weakness, nausea, vomiting, abdominal pain, fever
  - Hypotension from hypovolemia, impaired vascular response to catecholamines, loss of inotropic effects of cortisol
  - Altered mental status and confusion may be present
  - Hyperpigmentation of skin and mucous membranes in primary adrenal insufficiency
  - Hyponatremia, hyperkalemia, hypoglycemia, azotemia, hypercalcemia, eosinophilia, lymphocytosis
  - Serum cortisol >20 μg/dL makes diagnosis unlikely
  - ACTH stimulation test: increment of >7 μg/dL or peak cortisol level >17 μg/dL excludes adrenal insufficiency
  - Low to absent serum cortisol, elevated ACTH, abnormal ACTH simulation test in primary adrenal insufficiency
  - Suspect in anyone taking >30 mg of hydrocortisone per day (or equivalent) for more than 3 weeks in past 1 year
  - Etiologies of acute adrenal insufficiency: trauma; surgical stress; hemorrhage; infection; hypoperfusion; drugs; autoimmune; uncontrolled or poorly controlled chronic adrenal insufficiency with precipitating event

- **Differential Diagnosis**
  - Sepsis
  - Hypovolemia
  - Metastatic cancer
  - Salt wasting nephropathy
  - Medications
  - Acute abdomen
  - Secondary adrenal insufficiency: pituitary or hypothalamic disorders

- **Treatment**
  - Immediately treat with intravenous hydrocortisone when suspected; may use dexamethasone if ACTH stimulation test delayed
  - Add mineralocorticoid replacement with fludrocortisone if dexamethasone is used; not needed when >50 mg/d hydrocortisone administered
  - Correct hypovolemia and electrolyte abnormalities
  - Monitor and infuse glucose if hypoglycemic
  - May require vasopressors for blood pressure support
  - Consider empiric antibiotic therapy if infection suspected
  - Identify and treat precipitating event

- **Pearl**

Despite aggressive volume resuscitation and vasopressor use, patients with acute adrenal insufficiency may remain hypotensive until corticosteroid replacement has been administered.

Reference

Cooper MS et al: Corticosteroid insufficiency in acutely ill patients. N Engl J Med 2003;348:727. [PMID: 12594318]

Cushing Syndrome

- **Essentials of Diagnosis**
  - Weakness, proximal myopathy, weight gain, irregular menses, hirsutism, acne, neuropsychiatric problems
  - Plethoric moon facies, supraclavicular fullness, "buffalo hump," hypertension, cutaneous wasting, purple striae, poor wound healing, easy bruising
  - Insulin resistance, central obesity, hypertension, dyslipidemia, impaired glucose tolerance (similar to "metabolic syndrome")
  - Atherosclerosis, cardiovascular disease, nephrolithiasis, osteoporosis, polycystic ovary syndrome, hypogonadism
  - Hyperglycemia, glycosuria, leukocytosis, lymphocytopenia; possibly hypokalemia and metabolic alkalosis
  - Elevated levels of late-night serum and salivary cortisol levels or 24-hour urinary free cortisol levels
  - Overnight low-dose dexamethasone suppression test does not suppress plasma cortisol level
  - Consider dexamethasone-CRH test if above studies equivocal
  - Obtain ACTH levels once diagnosis of Cushing syndrome established
  - Additional tests may include pituitary or adrenal MRI or bilateral petrosal sinus ACTH sampling

- **Differential Diagnosis**
  - Metabolic syndrome
  - Obesity
  - Chronic alcoholism
  - Diabetes mellitus
  - Depression
  - Anorexia nervosa

- **Treatment**
  - Surgical removal of pituitary adenoma, adrenal tumor, or ectopic ACTH-producing tumor if present and resectable
  - Bilateral adrenalectomy for adrenal hyperplasia in refractory cases of ACTH-dependent Cushing syndrome
  - Ketoconazole or metyrapone to suppress cortisol production in unresectable cases

- **Pearl**

Cushing disease refers to manifestations of hypercortisolism due to pituitary hypersecretion of ACTH, while Cushing syndrome is produced by excessive exogenous corticosteroid use or excessive production from the adrenal cortex.

Reference

Raff HR et al: A physiologic approach to diagnosis of the Cushing syndrome. Ann Intern Med 2003;138:980. [PMID: 12809455]

Diabetic Ketoacidosis

- **Essentials of Diagnosis**
  - Polyuria, polydipsia, fatigue, weakness, weight loss, anorexia, nausea, vomiting, abdominal pain, lethargy
  - Marked volume depletion: decreased skin turgor, dry mucous membranes, sunken eyes, tachycardia, orthostatic hypotension
  - Deep rapid Kussmaul respirations; "fruity" odor on breath
  - Hypothermia unless precipitating event is infectious
  - Hyperglycemia >250 mg/dL, ketonemia, anion gap acidosis
  - Glycosuria, ketonuria, leukocytosis, hyperamylasemia, hyper-triglyceridemia; hyperkalemia despite depleted body stores
  - Serum osmolality variable; may be very high resulting in lethargy or coma
  - Typically occurs in younger lean patients with type 1 diabetes mellitus; increasingly seen in type 2; may be initial presentation
  - Precipitating event: infection, myocardial infarction, trauma, pancreatitis, medications, inadequate insulin

- **Differential Diagnosis**
  - Alcoholic ketoacidosis
  - Sepsis
  - Toxic ingestion
  - Starvation ketoacidosis
  - Lactic acidosis

- **Treatment**
  - Aggressive fluid replacement with normal saline; once glucose reaches 250–300 mg/dL add dextrose to infusion
  - Initial insulin bolus followed by intravenous insulin therapy (0.1 units/kg/h)
  - Replete potassium, phosphate, magnesium; begin potassium replacement immediately if initially normokalemic or hypokalemic
  - Frequent monitoring key to successful management: assessment of volume status especially in elderly or with cardiopulmonary disease; blood glucose every hour; electrolytes, renal function, ketones every 2–4 hours.
  - Identify and treat any precipitating event

- **Pearl**

A hyperchloremic non–gap metabolic acidosis is a common manifestation of the later treatment phase of diabetic ketoacidosis and takes longer to resolve than the gap ketoacidosis as its correction depends on the kidney's ability to regenerate bicarbonate.

Reference

Kitabchi AE et al: Hyperglycemic crises in patients with diabetes mellitus. Diabetes Care 2003;26:S109. [PMID: 12502633]

Hyperosmolar Non–ketotic Diabetic Coma

- **Essentials of Diagnosis**
  - Gradual onset of polyuria, polydipsia, polyphagia, fatigue, weakness, weight loss, anorexia, nausea, vomiting, altered mental status progressing to coma
  - Severe volume depletion: decreased skin turgor, dry mucous membranes, sunken eyes, tachycardia, orthostatic hypotension
  - Plasma glucose >600 mg/dL and serum osmolality >320 mOsm/kg; pH >7.3; absent or small amount of ketones; variable anion gap
  - Hypothermia common
  - Glycosuria, azotemia, leukocytosis
  - Risk factors: lack of prior knowledge of diabetes; older, obese patients with type 2 diabetes mellitus, underlying renal insufficiency, decreased access to water, female sex, underlying infection

- **Differential Diagnosis**
  - Diabetes insipidus: central or nephrogenic
  - Poorly controlled diabetes mellitus
  - Diabetic ketoacidosis
  - Toxic ingestion

- **Treatment**
  - Aggressive fluid replacement with normal saline (0.9% NaCl) to correct volume depletion; change to hypotonic fluid (0.45% NaCl or D_5 water) to reduce serum [Na^+] by 0.5–1.0 mEq/Lh
  - Once glucose reaches 300 mg/dL add dextrose to infusion
  - Goal glucose concentration should decrease by 100 mg/dL/h; may initiate intravenous insulin bolus and continuous insulin infusion but glucose may improve with hydration alone
  - Replete potassium, phosphate, magnesium; potassium loss is typically more severe than in diabetic ketoacidosis
  - Frequent monitoring key to successful management: assessment of volume status especially in elderly or with cardiopulmonary disease; blood glucose every hour; electrolytes, renal function, osmolality every 2–4 hours
  - Identify and treat any precipitating event

- **Pearl**

The lack of ketosis in hyperglycemic hyperosmolar non–ketotic coma may delay presentation resulting in ongoing osmotic diuresis that results in more severe volume depletion.

Reference

Kitabchi AE et al: Hyperglycemic crises in patients with diabetes mellitus. Diabetes Care 2003;26:S109. [PMID: 12502633]

Hypoglycemia

- ### Essentials of Diagnosis
  - Plasma glucose <45 mg/dL
  - Sweating, trembling, feeling of warmth, palpitations, anxiety, nausea, hunger, blurred or double vision, weakness
  - Neuroglycopenic symptoms with prolonged hypoglycemia: dizziness, confusion, tiredness, difficulty speaking, headache, inability to concentrate, nightmares, bizarre behavior
  - Clinical diagnostic criteria for insulinoma (Whipple triad): hypoglycemic symptoms in fasting or exercising state, low plasma glucose level, relief of symptoms through correction of hypoglycemia
  - Insulin and C-peptide levels may help determine cause
  - In nondiabetic hospitalized patients common etiologies include renal insufficiency, malnutrition, liver disease, infection, sepsis
  - Other causes: alcoholism, adrenal insufficiency, medications (insulin, sulfonylurea, pentamidine, trimethoprim-sulfamethoxazole, salicylates, beta-blocking agents), insulin-secreting tumors

- ### Differential Diagnosis
  - Delirium
  - Pheochromocytoma
  - Factitious hypoglycemia
  - Liver failure
  - Psychoneurosis
  - Sepsis syndrome
  - Myxedema coma

- ### Treatment
  - Administer glucose intravenously or orally (if awake and alert)
  - Monitor blood glucose closely as patient may need continuous dextrose infusion until precipitating cause removed
  - Glucagon and hydrocortisone can be given for refractory hypoglycemia
  - Identify and treat underlying disease or remove causative agent

- ### Pearl
Because the liver and kidneys are the primary organs involved in the metabolism of insulin and the sulfonylurea drugs, development of renal or hepatic failure may delay drug clearance and result in hypoglycemia.

Reference

Service FL: Hypoglycemic disorders. N Engl J Med 1995;332:1144. [PMID: 7700289]

Myxedema Coma

- **Essentials of Diagnosis**
  - Cold intolerance, weight gain, constipation, depression, menstrual irregularities
  - Puffy expressionless face; dry, rough, cold skin; non–pitting doughy edema; loss of eyebrows and scalp hair; delayed relaxation phase of tendon reflexes; enlarged tongue; bladder distention; decreased gastrointestinal motility
  - Hypothermia, bradycardia, elevated diastolic blood pressure
  - Hypercapnic respiratory failure with hypoxemia
  - Altered mental status: confusion, somnolence, coma
  - Low T_4 and T_3, low T_3 resin uptake, elevated TSH
  - Hypoglycemia, hyponatremia, anemia, elevated creatine phosphokinase, elevated creatinine, hyperlipidemia
  - Radiographs may reveal enlarged cardiac silhouette, pleural and pericardial effusions
  - ECG findings: bradycardia, low voltage, diffuse T wave depression, nonspecific ST changes, prolonged QT and PR intervals, conduction blocks
  - Risk factors: known hypothyroidism with absent or inadequate thyroid replacement and precipitating stress or illness

- **Differential Diagnosis**
  - Primary amyloidosis
  - Toxic ingestion
  - Obstructive sleep apnea, obesity hypoventilation syndrome
  - Exposure hypothermia
  - Parkinson disease

- **Treatment**
  - Intravenous T_4 until able to tolerate oral therapy; decrease dose in frail patients or with significant cardiac disease
  - Intravenous glucocorticoids until adrenal insufficiency excluded by cortisol level or ACTH stimulation test
  - Correct hypothermia, hypovolemia, electrolyte abnormalities
  - May require mechanical ventilation for hypoventilation
  - Medication dose adjustment given impaired drug clearance with severe hypothyroidism
  - Identify and treat precipitating event

- **Pearl**

In patients with hypothyroidism, the manifestations of adrenal insufficiency may be masked. If in doubt, administer glucocorticoids concomitantly with levothyroxine therapy to avoid precipitating adrenal crisis.

Reference

Ringel MD: Management of hypothyroidism and hyperthyroidism in the intensive care unit. Crit Care Clin 2001;17:59. [PMID 11219235]

| **Sick Euthyroid Syndrome** |

- **Essentials of Diagnosis**
  - Low T_3 in clinically euthyroid patients with acute or chronic nonthyroidal illness; reverse T_3 may be increased; free T4 almost always normal; can be reduced in prolonged severe illness
  - Normal TSH indicate "euthyroid state"
  - TSH > 20 μU/mL in sick individuals suggestive of primary hypothyroidism
  - TSH < 0.1 μU/mL may be hyperthyroidism or sick euthyroid syndrome; differentiate by thyrotropin-releasing hormone stimulation test: sick euthyroid patients show detectable responses of TSH, hyperthyroid have absent response
  - Very common; may affect up to 70% of hospitalized patients; complex, multifaceted response of endocrine system to illness
  - Medications may affect thyroid function: dopamine, high-dose corticosteroids, and octreotide suppress TSH secretion; amiodarone results in low T_3 and normal or elevated T_4; propranolol, metoprolol, atenolol in large doses decrease T_3; rifampin increases T_4 clearance

- **Differential Diagnosis**
  - Primary hypothyroidism
  - Secondary hypothyroidism
  - Diabetes mellitus
  - Renal disease
  - Acute myocardial infarction
  - Malnutrition/caloric deprivation
  - AIDS
  - Chronic liver disease
  - Cancer
  - Infection
  - Surgery
  - Medications

- **Treatment**
  - Supportive measures: adequate nutrition; specific and successful treatment of underlying illness should result in normalization of thyroid function abnormalities
  - Replacing T_3 and T_4 have not demonstrated mortality benefits; animal studies suggest increased mortality with T_3 and T_4 replacement

- **Pearl**

In prolonged critical illness, the fall in T_3 is accompanied by a fall in T_4 and portends a poor outcome. In patients with a T_4 concentration <3 μg/dL mortality rates reach as high as 80%.

Reference

Vasa FR et al: Endocrine problems in the chronically critically ill patient. Clin Chest Med 2001;1:193. [PMID 11315456]

Thyroid Storm

- **Essentials of Diagnosis**
  - Heat intolerance, nervousness, increased number of bowel movements, increased appetite, weight loss, thinning of hair and skin, sweating, weakness
  - Confusion, agitation, overt psychosis, coma
  - Fever due to breakdown of thermoregulatory system
  - Cardiovascular manifestations: tachycardia, atrial fibrillation, hypertension, widened pulse pressure, congestive heart failure; hypotension late manifestation
  - Ophthalmopathy, dermopathy, thyroid bruit with Graves disease
  - Warm, moist, flushed, soft "velvety" skin; tremor; brisk tendon reflexes; proximal myopathy; generalized cachexia
  - Goiter almost always present
  - Elevated T_4 and T_3 typically seen; nearly undetectable TSH
  - Elevated aminotransferases, hyperbilirubinemia, alkaline phosphatase (bone fraction), calcium
  - Uncontrolled or poorly controlled hyperthyroidism with precipitating event: surgical procedure, infection, cardiovascular disease, diabetic ketoacidosis, stroke, trauma, anesthesia, administration of iodinated contrast material

- **Differential Diagnosis**
  - Sepsis
  - Acute psychiatric illness
  - Toxic ingestion
  - Pheochromocytoma
  - Levothyroxine overdose
  - Alcohol withdrawal

- **Treatment**
  - Identify and treat precipitating event
  - Reduce thyroid hormone synthesis or peripheral conversion of T_4 to T_3 using thiourea (propylthiouracil or methimazole) followed by ipodate sodium (iodine-containing contrast agent)
  - Inhibit release of thyroid hormone with iodide (sodium iodide or Lugol solution); lithium if intolerant of iodine
  - Sympathetic blockade with propranolol; also weakly inhibits peripheral conversion of T_4 to T_3
  - Glucocorticoids inhibit TSH secretion, lower T_4 levels; also use in those with suspected adrenal insufficiency
  - Correct hyperthermia, hypovolemia, electrolyte abnormalities

- **Pearl**

Avoid salicylates in the management of hyperthermia in thyroid storm as they can displace thyroid hormone from its binding sites and worsen this hyperthyroid state.

Reference

Tietgens ST et al: Thyroid storm. Med Clin North Am 1995;79:169. [PMID: 7808090]

13

Neurology

Altered Mental Status in the ICU

- **Essentials of Diagnosis**
  - Agitation, delirium, decreased sensorium, or waxing and waning of consciousness
  - Disorganized thinking with rambling, incoherent speech, shouting, moaning
  - Hallucinations or illusions; appear fearful, restless
  - Disorientation to time, place, situation
  - Serial examinations imperative as symptoms may fluctuate
  - Agitated patients can demonstrate hypertension, tachycardia, tachypnea, increased oxygen needs, ventilatory difficulties
  - Difficult to assess pharmacologically sedated patients
  - Mini Mental Status Examination (MMSE), Cognitive Test for Delirium (CTD), Confusion Assessment Method for the Intensive Care Unit (CAM-ICU) may be helpful
  - Dementia and delirium may be differentiated by EEG findings
  - Delirium in ICU associated with increased mortality, length of stay, need for subsequent nursing home placement

- **Differential Diagnosis**
  - Hypoxemia, hypoperfusion
  - Hypoglycemia, electrolyte abnormalities
  - Thyrotoxicosis
  - Postoperative states
  - Sleep deprivation, head trauma
  - Postictal states
  - Medications, withdrawal or intoxication
  - Infection: systemic, CNS, HIV

- **Treatment**
  - Identify causes, withdraw potential offending drugs, treat underlying etiology
  - Symptomatic treatment if patient is danger to self or others
  - Enlist assistance from family to aid in orientation to self, location, time (day/night), situation
  - If unexplained, consider trial of benzodiazepines to exclude alcohol or benzodiazepine withdrawal; haloperidol with or without a benzodiazepine; or atypical antipsychotic

- **Pearl**

Instructing patients to report strange phenomenon, empathetically informing them you understand their sense of confusion, and reassuring family members are important aspects of the social and psychologic management of ICU patients.

Reference

Cohen IL et al: Management of the agitated intensive care unit patient. Crit Care Med 2003;30:S97. [PMID: 11852874]

Critical Illness Myopathy

- **Essentials of Diagnosis**
  - Weakness of extremities or respiratory muscles without sensory deficit; no evidence of neuropathy, spinal cord, central nervous system disorders
  - Rarely elevated creatine kinase or aldolase unless necrotizing component
  - May occur with or without critical illness polyneuropathy
  - Electromyogram insensitive; muscle biopsy may be useful
  - Probably caused by cytokine-induced effects on muscle protein; potential mediators include IL-1, TNF
  - Myopathy with prolonged weakness frequent complication of corticosteroids plus non-depolarizing neuromuscular blockers

- **Differential Diagnosis**
  - Primary muscle disorders: polymyositis, dermatomyositis
  - Steroid myopathy
  - Prolonged effects of non–depolarizing muscle relaxants
  - Alcoholic myopathy
  - Malnutrition
  - Drugs: statins, nucleoside reverse transcriptase inhibitor, colchicine, vincristine
  - Electrolyte abnormalities: hypokalemia, hypophosphatemia
  - Hypo- and hyperthyroidism

- **Treatment**
  - No specific treatment; correct underlying sepsis or organ failure
  - Discontinue potentially myopathic medications; correct electrolyte abnormalities
  - Most have slow spontaneous improvement; recovery may be limited or absent if severe
  - Weakness may persist long after critical illness resolves

- **Pearl**

Corticosteroids plus non–depolarizing neuromuscular blockers cause a synergistic myopathy with severe prolonged weakness; avoid if possible.

Reference

Deem S et al: Acquired neuromuscular disorders in the intensive care unit. Am J Respir Crit Care Med 2003;168:735. [PMID: 14522811]

Critical Illness Polyneuropathy

■ Essentials of Diagnosis
- Flaccid weakness, loss of reflexes, sensory deficits indicating peripheral neuropathy
- Consider with weakness, failure to wean, decreased sensation in extremities
- Up to 70% of sepsis or multiorgan failure, especially with prolonged ICU stay
- Distal axonopathy, degeneration of axons without inflammation due to neuropathic consequence of decreased perfusion; no evidence of nutritional deficiency, neuritis, drug effects
- Nerve conduction studies: reduced muscle and sensory action potentials, fibrillations, loss of motor unit potentials with maximal effort; no slowing of nerve conduction, conduction blocks, demyelination

■ Differential Diagnosis
- Guillain-Barré syndrome
- Botulism
- Myasthenia gravis
- Prolonged effects of non-depolarizing muscle relaxants
- Malnutrition
- Paraneoplastic syndromes
- Myopathies, including critical illness myopathy, corticosteroids, hypokalemia

■ Treatment
- No specific treatment; correct underlying sepsis or organ failure; discontinue potentially neuropathic and myopathic medications (isoniazid, aminoglycosides, vincristine, corticosteroids); correct electrolyte abnormalities
- Treat for vitamin deficiency (pyridoxine, thiamine)
- Most have slow spontaneous improvement; recovery may be limited or absent if severe

■ Pearl
Critical illness polyneuropathy should be considered in any patient who is difficult to wean from mechanical ventilation.

Reference
Hund E: Critical illness polyneuropathy. Curr Opin Neurol 2001;14:649. [PMID: 11562578]

Guillain-Barré Syndrome

- **Essentials of Diagnosis**
  - Acute or subacute ascending progressive symmetric flaccid paralysis with antecedent flulike syndrome or vaccination
  - Paresthesias and pain; sensory symptoms mild or absent; occasional cranial nerve deficits; autonomic dysfunction variable
  - Areflexia occurs early; pupils and eyelids spared
  - Lumbar puncture demonstrates "albuminocytologic dissociation" (elevated protein without pleocytosis); can be diagnostic by second week
  - Electromyogram: segmental demyelination, reduction of velocity (AIDP) or axonal injury (AMSAN and AMAN)
  - Spectrum of disease: acute inflammatory demyelinating polyradiculopathy (AIDP), acute motor-sensory axonal neuropathy (AMSAN), acute motor-axonal neuropathy (AMAN), Miller-Fisher syndrome
  - Etiologies: idiopathic most common; infection with *Campylobacter jejuni*, *Mycoplasma pneumonia*, CMV, EBV, VZV, Hepatitis B
  - Risks for persistent disability: progression to quadriparesis in <7 days, need for ventilatory support, mean distal motor amplitude <20% lower limits of normal, age >60
  - Recovery typically begins 2–4 wk after progression stops

- **Differential Diagnosis**
  - Poliomyelitis, myasthenia gravis, botulism, Lambert-Eaton syndrome, diphtheria, transverse myelitis
  - Periodic paralysis   • Heavy metal toxicity
  - Porphyria

- **Treatment**
  - Monitor vital capacity (VC); intubation may be needed if VC <15 mL/kg or to protect against aspiration
  - Monitor for sinus tachycardia; asystole may occur
  - Opiates for pain control, adequate nutrition, bowel care, psychological support
  - Plasma exchange or high-dose intravenous immunoglobulin

- **Pearl**

More than one third of patients with Guillain-Barré syndrome will require ICU admission for respiratory failure, dysautonomia, or other complications.

Reference

Hahn AF: Guillain-Barré syndrome. Lancet 1998;352:635. [PMID: 9746040]

Head Injuries

- **Essentials of Diagnosis**
  - Manifestations depend on extent and location of injury: asymptomatic; headache, nausea, vomiting, or amnesia; lethargy, increased somnolence, transient loss of consciousness, confusion, or unresponsiveness; papilledema, pupillary changes, Battle sign, "raccoon eyes," or focal neurologic signs
  - Primary injuries include skull fracture, concussion, cerebral contusion, intracranial hemorrhage, diffuse axonal injury
  - Secondary injuries include intracranial insults (intracranial hypertension, herniation, cerebral ischemia or infarction); systemic insults (hypoxia, hypotension, electrolyte imbalances)
  - Complete neurological examination including Glasgow Coma Scale and brain stem function
  - CT scan diagnostic; cerebral angiography identifies dissection, traumatic pseudoaneurysm, vasospasm
  - Assess for concomitant spinal injury; occurs in 6–8%

- **Differential Diagnosis**
  - Seizure, stroke, brain tumor
  - Hypoglycemia, neurosyphilis
  - Vasculitis

- **Treatment**
  - Stabilize spine
  - Monitor and protect airway; intubation indicated if GCS < 8; fiberoptic guidance for intubation in cervical spine injuries
  - Monitor cardiac rhythm; fluid resuscitation for SBP < 110 mm Hg; avoid hypotonic solutions
  - Serial neurologic examination to monitor for decompensation
  - Stabilize with target $PaCO_2$ 35–40 mm Hg, mean arterial blood pressure $\geq$ 90 mm Hg, normal intravascular volume and electrolytes
  - Manage elevated intracranial pressure: monitor with ventriculostomy; removal of CSF, short-term hyperventilation, head elevation, sedation, correction of hyperthermia; barbiturate coma if maximal medical therapy failed
  - Surgical indications: failing medical management; prevent irreversible damage if neurologically deteriorating; certain contusions, hematomas, foreign bodies

- **Pearl**

Improved outcomes associated with head trauma are due in part to early recognition and prevention of disorders that cause secondary brain injury.

Reference

Guidelines for the management of severe head injury, 2nd ed. Brain Trauma Foundation, 2000.

Increased Intracranial Pressure

- **Essentials of Diagnosis**
  - Headache; nausea or vomiting; depressed level of consciousness
  - Abnormal pupillary response; cranial nerve deficits (particularly CN VI); papilledema; abnormal posturing; hypo- or hyperventilation; focal neurologic deficits or abnormal reflexes
  - Cushing triad: hypertension, bradycardia, abnormal respirations (late finding)
  - CT scan or MRI: intracranial bleed, mass, midline shift, edema, decreased size of ventricles or basilar cistern, effacement of sulci
  - Direct measurement of ICP diagnostic
  - Etiologies: head trauma, intracranial hemorrhage, meningitis/meningoencephalitis, malignancy (primary or metastatic), osmotic changes, hydrocephalus

- **Differential Diagnosis**
  - Meningitis/meningoencephalitis, stroke, encephalopathy
  - Intoxication, nutritional deficiency

- **Treatment**
  - Intubate for altered mental status and to control Pa_{CO_2}
  - Monitor cardiac rhythm; adequate intravenous access; correct hypovolemia; avoid hypotonic solutions
  - Elevate head of bed 15–30°
  - Mannitol for acute management; monitor serum osmolarity
  - Hyperventilation for acute management; once stabilized, taper over 6–12 hours; avoid profound hyperventilation (keep Pa_{CO_2} 30–35 mm Hg)
  - Sedate with opioids, benzodiazepines, propofol to lower chance of increasing ICP during suctioning, coughing, repositioning; paralytic agents mask changes in neurologic exam
  - Remove cerebrospinal fluid or intracranial mass lesion
  - Corticosteroids only useful in malignancy, abscess, postneurosurgical procedure
  - Correct hyperthermia; induced hypothermia controversial
  - Pentobarbital used if other maneuvers fail; monitor for hypotension

- **Pearl**

Small changes in intracranial volume may cause intracranial pressure to increase because of the inelastic properties of the skull.

Reference

Allen CH et al: An evidence-based approach to management of increased intracranial pressure. Crit Care Clin 1998;14:485. [PMID: 9700443]

Muscular Dystrophy

■ Essentials of Diagnosis

- Progressive muscle wasting and weakness
- Typically proximal muscle involvement; pseudohypertrophy of gastrocnemius muscle
- Mental impairment common in Duchenne muscular dystrophy
- Elevated creatine kinase
- Characteristic electromyogram and electrocardiogram: tall right precordial R wave and precordial Q waves
- Muscle biopsy: fiber necrosis, size variation, infiltration by macrophages; replacement by connective tissue and fat
- Pulmonary complications include respiratory insufficiency and infection; cardiac complications include cardiomyopathy and conduction system abnormalities
- Inherited myogenic disorders: congenital, Duchenne and Becker, Emery-Dreifuss, distal, facioscapulohumeral, oculopharyngeal
- Increase rate of adverse events to anesthetics

■ Differential Diagnosis

- Dermatopolymyositis
- Myasthenia gravis
- Amyotrophic lateral sclerosis
- Botulism
- Guillain-Barré syndrome
- Lambert-Eaton syndrome

■ Treatment

- No proven treatment currently available
- Monitor and manage complications
- Consider noninvasive ventilatory support for respiratory insufficiency; elective intubation if vital capacity <15– 20 mL/kg; tracheostomy for prolonged support
- Cardiomyopathy treated with standard medications; pacemaker or defibrillator for conduction system defects and arrhythmias

■ Pearl

Because of the risk of rhabdomyolysis, myoglobinuria, acceleration of muscle weakness, and hyperkalemic cardiac arrest, avoid succinylcholine in patients with Duchenne or Becker muscular dystrophy.

Reference

Emery AE: The muscular dystrophies. Lancet 2002;359:687. [PMID: 11879882]

Myasthenia Gravis

- **Essentials of Diagnosis**
  - Painless, fluctuating weakness; pronounced in proximal muscles
  - Ptosis and diplopia; reduced facial expression; weakness in speaking and chewing muscles; dysphagia
  - Reflexes and sensory examination normal
  - Weakness evident with tests of fatigue: repetitive shoulder abduction or upward gaze
  - Acetylcholine receptor antibodies found in 85–90%
  - Edrophonium (Tensilon) test yields improved motor function
  - Nerve conduction studies demonstrate decremental response
  - CT or MRI to evaluate for thymoma
  - Associated conditions: thymoma, thyroid disease, polymyositis, rheumatoid arthritis, systemic lupus erythematosus
  - Myasthenic crisis precipitated by infections; trauma or surgery; medications including antiarrhythmics, antibiotics, antihypertensives, sedatives, paralytics

- **Differential Diagnosis**
  - Botulism
  - Lambert-Eaton syndrome
  - Toxins
  - Guillain-Barré syndrome
  - Myopathies
  - Cholinergic crisis

- **Treatment**
  - Monitor pulmonary function with vital capacity; ventilatory support when vital capacity <15–20 mL/kg
  - Anticholinesterase inhibitor: pyridostigmine
  - Corticosteroids and other immunosuppressive therapy
  - Plasma exchange or intravenous immune globulin if no response
  - Thymectomy for young aged onset, AChR antibody–positive, generalized symptoms
  - Monitor cardiac status as risk for atrial fibrillation, ventricular fibrillation, asystole
  - Discontinue any medications and treat any infection that could worsen crisis
  - Ensure adequate nutrition, bowel care, psychological support

- **Pearl**

During an exacerbation, management is dependent on differentiating myasthenic crisis from cholinergic crisis (hypersalivation, lacrimation, miosis, vomiting, and sweating).

Reference

Vincent A et al: Myasthenia gravis. Lancet 2001;357:2122. [PMID: 11445126]

Neuroleptic Malignant Syndrome

- Essentials of Diagnosis
  - Hyperthermia and muscle rigidity related to use of phenothiazines, butyrophenones, thioxanthenes, benzamides and other postsynaptic dopamine blockers; atypical neuroleptics implicated in case reports
  - Mental status varies from agitation or confusion to coma; encephalopathy
  - Autonomic dysfunction including diaphoresis, tachycardia, hypertension, tachypnea, urinary incontinence
  - Extrapyramidal signs such as tremor, cog-wheel rigidity, dystonia, dyskinesis, chorea, opisthotonos, opsoclonus, posturing
  - Granulocytosis, hyperglycemia, elevated creatine kinase, elevated serum catecholamines
  - Complications: pulmonary edema, ischemic bowel, paralytic ileus; rhabdomyolysis due to "lead pipe rigidity" of muscles
  - Increased risk: organic brain disease, affective illnesses, dehydration, alcoholism, sympathoadrenal hyperactivity

- Differential Diagnosis
  - Malignant hyperthermia
  - Central anticholinergic syndrome
  - Thyrotoxicosis
  - Lethal catatonia
  - Encephalitis/meningitis
  - Heat stroke
  - Pheochromocytoma
  - Toxins: cocaine, methamphetamines, tricyclic antidepressants with lithium or monoamine oxidase inhibitors, metoclopramide, or reserpine

- Treatment
  - Discontinue and avoid dopamine-blocking agents
  - Cooling measures
  - Aggressive intravenous crystalloid infusion to stabilize hemodynamics and prevent or treat rhabdomyolysis
  - Bromocriptine and dantrolene to control rigidity and high temperature; amantadine and levodopa-carbidopa can reduce hyperthermia
  - Continue treatment 2–3 wk until symptoms resolve
  - Recurrence common; rechallenge with lower potency medications at lower doses if necessary

- Pearl

Differentiate malignant hyperthermia from neuroleptic malignant syndrome by lack of encephalopathy or autonomic dysfunction.

Reference

Adnet P et al: Neuroleptic malignant syndrome. Br J Anaesth 2000;85:129.
   [PMID: 10928001]

Seizures

- **Essentials of Diagnosis**
  - Abrupt onset tonic-clonic activity, focal twitching, eye movements, blinking, confusion, or unresponsiveness
  - Simple partial seizures arise from focal area without alteration of consciousness
  - Complex partial seizures arise from temporal lobe; autonomic or emotional symptoms, déjà vu or hallucinations; altered consciousness with motionless stare or lip smacking
  - Generalized tonic-clonic seizures may start with outburst followed by tonic then rhythmic clonic phase involving all extremities; associated with loss of consciousness
  - Absence seizures begin abruptly with loss of contact; occasional eye fluttering, maintenance of body tone followed by abrupt recovery; no postictal state
  - Status epilepticus: persistence of seizure >10 min or incomplete recovery between seizures
  - EEG diagnostic if obtained during or soon after seizure
  - CT scan to assess for structural disease
  - Lumbar puncture if infection suspected

- **Differential Diagnosis**
  - Hypoxic-ischemic event
  - Encephalitis
  - Drug withdrawal
  - Metabolic encephalopathies
  - Structural brain injury
  - Psychiatric disease
  - Medication toxicity

- **Treatment**
  - Identify and treat precipitating cause
  - Acutely control with benzodiazepines or other anticonvulsants
  - Stabilize hemodynamics; ensure adequate intravenous access
  - Infuse thiamine and glucose empirically
  - Laboratory evaluation: arterial blood gas, metabolic panel, glucose, toxicologic screen, drug levels, complete blood count
  - Status epilepticus: administer intravenous phenytoin; if uncontrolled after 20–30 min intubate and add intravenous phenobarbital; if persistent after 40–60 min add continuous infusion of pentobarbital, midazolam, or propofol with continuous EEG monitoring

- **Pearl**

Although CSF pleocytosis occurs, exclude other causes such as meningitis before attributing this finding to status epilepticus.

Reference

Sirven JI et al: Management of status epilepticus. Am Fam Physician 2003;68:469. [PMID: 12924830]

Spinal Cord Compression

■ Essentials of Diagnosis

- Axial pain early symptom with localized tenderness over involved spinal segment; thoracic (70%), lumbar (20%), cervical (10%) involvement
- Presentation depends on location of lesion: weakness; tingling or numbness; urinary retention; bowel or bladder incontinence
- Motor impairment can begin distally; tendon reflexes may be increased and Babinski sign may be present
- Sensory impairment may manifest as sensory level
- CSF examination typically not helpful
- Radiographs may demonstrate vertebral body collapse or destruction, loss of pedicles
- Obtain emergent MRI; CT myelography if MRI not available
- Biopsy for suspected infections or if primary tumor unknown
- Etiologies: abscesses, hematoma, disk fragments in spinal canal, tumors including lung, breast, prostate, lymphoma, multiple myeloma
- Infectious agents include: cysticercosis, *Staphylococcus aureus*, *Mycobacterium tuberculosis*, anaerobes, varicella-zoster virus, polio virus

■ Differential Diagnosis

- Disk herniation
- Benign neoplasms
- Transverse myelitis
- Paraneoplastic syndromes
- Vascular disease
- Neurologic disorders
- Leptomeningeal carcinomatosis

■ Treatment

- Appropriate antibiotics for infectious etiologies
- Neurosurgical consultation indicated for all other etiologies
- Initiate corticosteroids prior to obtaining formal studies in cases of suspected malignancy; localized radiation therapy and tumor-specific chemotherapy if malignancy is confirmed
- In metastatic disease, laminectomy or surgical decompression for spinal instability, no response to radiation therapy, previous XRT up to cord tolerance, high cervical or atlantoaxial disease, radioresistant tumor, solitary metastasis

■ Pearl

Vertebral metastases rarely cross the disk space, unlike infectious causes.

Reference

Daw HA et al: Epidural spinal cord compression in cancer patients: diagnosis and management. Cleve Clin J Med 2000;67:497. [PMID: 10902239]

Spinal Cord Injury

- **Essentials of Diagnosis**
  - Incomplete injuries: anterior cord syndrome with loss of motor function, pain and temperature, normal proprioception and vibration; central cord syndrome with motor and sensory findings in distal upper extremities >lower; posterior column syndrome with loss of vibration, proprioception, discrimination; Brown-Séquard syndrome with loss of ipsilateral motor and dorsal column function, contralateral loss of pain and temperature sensation one or two levels below injury
  - Damage to upper and lower motor neurons accompanies almost all cases
  - Assess for brain and multilevel injury
  - Radiographs to assess prevertebral soft tissue swelling, alignment, angulation of spinal canal, fractures; dynamic views contraindicated with acute neurological dysfunction
  - MRI for neurological symptoms with negative plain radiographs
  - CT scan for evaluation of fracture or subluxation, poorly visualized areas, or if MRI contraindicated

- **Differential Diagnosis**
  - Amyotrophic lateral sclerosis, multiple sclerosis, transverse myelitis
  - Aortic dissection, primary or metastatic cancer

- **Treatment**
  - Stabilize spine; monitor and protect airway; oxygen and aggressive pulmonary toilet; fiberoptic guided intubation if cervical spine injuries
  - Intravenous fluids typically improve hypotension from spinal shock; monitor and treat cardiac arrhythmias; atropine or pacemaker for bradycardia
  - Assess neurologic examination serially for decompensation
  - High dose methylprednisolone within 3–8 hours of injury
  - Surgery indicated for: decompression of incompletely injured neural tissue, reduction and stabilization of malaligned or unstable cervical segments
  - Nasogastric tube, Foley catheter for atonic GI tract, bladder

- **Pearl**

Depolarizing neuromuscular blocking agents may lead to hyperkalemia and ventricular fibrillation in patients with spinal cord injuries.

Reference

McDonald JW et al: Spinal cord injury. Lancet 2002;359:417. [PMID: 11844532]

Stroke

- **■ Essentials of Diagnosis**
  - Signs depend on location and include hemiplegia, hemiparesis, hemisensory loss, aphasia, cranial nerve abnormalities, hemianopia, impaired cerebellar function, impaired cortical function, dysarthria
  - Sudden neurologic symptoms reaching maximal deficit at onset seen with acute embolic strokes
  - Acute hemorrhagic stroke with sudden onset; likelihood of hemorrhage increases with coma, vomiting, severe headache, systolic blood pressure >220 mm Hg, warfarin use
  - Sudden onset followed by stepwise or progressive involvement seen with occlusive vascular disease
  - Head CT scan insensitive in first 24 hours if bland infarct; very sensitive for hemorrhagic stroke
  - MRI may have higher sensitivity in early ischemic stroke; MR angiography useful for evaluating occlusive disease
  - Risk factors: hypertension, diabetes, smoking, cardiovascular disease, atrial fibrillation, valvular heart disease, family history of premature cardiovascular disease

- **■ Differential Diagnosis**
  - Seizure
  - Neurosyphilis
  - Subdural or epidural hematoma
  - Hypoglycemia
  - Brain tumor
  - Vasculitis

- **■ Treatment**
  - Stabilize and protect airway; ensure adequate intravenous access; monitor and treat cardiac arrhythmias
  - Optimal blood pressure control not clear; cautious use of parenteral medication for SBP > 220 mm Hg or DBP > 120 mm Hg
  - Assess neurologic examination serially for decompensation
  - Aspirin given within 24–48 hours
  - Tissue plasminogen activator (r-tPA) for carefully selected patients with ischemic stroke treated within 3 h of onset; intra-arterial thrombolysis may be helpful
  - Correct abnormalities such as hypoglycemia or hyponatremia

- **■ Pearl**

Hypotension or rapid decreases in blood pressure should be avoided because autoregulation of cerebral blood flow is impaired and regional brain perfusion is dependent upon systemic blood pressure.

Reference

Adams HP et al: Guidelines for the early management of patients with ischemic stroke. Stroke 2003;34:1056. [PMID: 12677087]

Stupor & Coma

- **Essentials of Diagnosis**
  - Patient unresponsive to any stimuli
  - Develops as result of diffuse dysfunction of cerebral cortices or injury to reticular activating system
  - Diencephalon lesions: 1- to 2-mm pupils, normal eye movements, flexion abnormalities, Cheyne-Stokes respirations
  - Midbrain lesions: fixed and midline pupils, disconjugate eye movements, extension abnormalities, hyperventilation
  - Pontine lesions: coma, pinpoint pupils, paralysis of extraocular muscles, extension abnormalities, hyperventilation
  - Medullary lesions: variable mental status, pupil size, and eye movements; flaccid muscles, apnea, circulatory collapse
  - Assess level of consciousness with Glasgow Coma Score; check for nuchal rigidity; asymmetry in neurologic examination; funduscopic examination
  - Laboratory studies helpful for etiology or monitoring: metabolic panel, arterial blood gas, toxicologic screen, serum osmolality, serum medication levels
  - CT or MRI of brain; LP if possible infection; EEG if seizure suspected
  - Etiologies: metabolic, toxic, structural brain injury

- **Differential Diagnosis**
  - Seizure/postictal state, brainstem herniation
  - Hypertensive encephalopathy, catatonia
  - Hypercapnia/hypoventilation syndrome
  - Increased intracranial pressure

- **Treatment**
  - Protect airway; indications for intubation: absent gag reflex, respiratory compromise, control of $Paco_2$ to aid in management of intracranial hypertension
  - Avoid sudden drops in blood pressure as this may result in herniation or irreversible brain injury
  - Intravenous thiamine followed by dextrose and naloxone; consider empiric antibiotics if diagnosis of meningitis or encephalitis entertained

- **Pearl**

Under no circumstances should the pupils in a comatose patient be dilated to aid with retinal examination since changes in the pupil size are often the most reliable clinical indication of deterioration following acute brain injury.

Reference

Liao YJ et al: An approach to critically ill patients in coma. West J Med 2002;176:184. [PMID: 12016243]

Subarachnoid Hemorrhage (SAH)

- ■ Essentials of Diagnosis
  - Symptoms preceded days or weeks by headache from sentinel leak followed by "thunderclap" headache: sudden onset, reaching maximal intensity in minutes, "worst headache of their life"
  - Nausea, vomiting, photophobia, neck stiffness or pain
  - Nuchal rigidity, papilledema, retinal hemorrhages, nystagmus
  - Neurologic deficits depend on location and severity of bleed: cranial nerve palsies, aphasia, hemiparesis, neglect
  - Subarachnoid blood on CT scan in first 48 hours
  - Perform lumbar puncture when CT scan negative but history suggestive; bloody or xanthochromic fluid sensitive finding
  - Obtain four-vessel cerebral angiogram once SAH diagnosed: localizes aneurysm, defines anatomy, identifies vasospasm
  - Associated diseases: hypertension, polycystic kidney disease, Ehlers-Danlos syndrome, arteriovenous malformations, pseudoxanthoma elasticum, coarctation of aorta
  - Complications: rebleeding, vasospasm, hydrocephalus

- ■ Differential Diagnosis
  - Meningitis/encephalitis
  - Increased intracranial pressure
  - Tension headache
  - Stroke
  - Temporal arteritis
  - Migraine headache

- ■ Treatment
  - Monitor and protect airway; intubate comatose individuals and patients with respiratory compromise
  - Stabilize hemodynamics: adequate intravenous access; tight blood pressure control avoiding hypotension or hypertension; transfuse to correct coagulopathy or thrombocytopenia
  - Supportive therapy: avoid stress or straining, maintain at bed rest in quiet setting, analgesics for pain control
  - Early intervention with surgical clips or embolization
  - Vasospasm prophylaxis with calcium channel blocker nimodipine
  - Seizure prophylaxis with phenytoin
  - Correct electrolyte abnormalities, especially hyponatremia

- ■ Pearl

Vasospasm, a potentially devastating complication of SAH, can be managed with "Triple H" therapy (induced hypervolemia, hemodilution, and hypertension), which augments cerebral blood flow and prevents ischemic cellular damage.

Reference

Edlow JA et al: Avoiding pitfalls in the diagnosis of subarachnoid hemorrhage. N Engl J Med 2000;342:29. [PMID: 10620647]

14

Renal Disorders

Acute Tubular Necrosis (ATN)

- **Essentials of Diagnosis**
  - Acute renal failure without prerenal, postrenal, glomerular, or interstitial features
  - History of hypotension, exposure to nephrotoxic antibiotics or radiocontrast agents
  - Reduced urine output, malaise, nausea, altered sensorium
  - Acute onset oliguria with ischemic ATN; $Fe_{Na} > 1\%$ but may be nonoliguric
  - Urinalysis: muddy brown granular casts, epithelial cells, red cells, white cells; unremarkable sediment in toxin-induced ATN
  - Inability of kidney to regulate sodium, electrolytes, water
  - Usually in conjunction with multiorgan failure, ARDS, medications
  - Leading cause of acute renal failure in ICU; mortality rate 50–80% among those requiring dialysis

- **Differential Diagnosis**
  - Sepsis
  - Hypoperfusion or ischemia
  - Radiocontrast media administration
  - Medications: aminoglycosides, amphotericin B, cisplatin
  - Myoglobinuria and hemoglobinuria

- **Treatment**
  - Prevention: N-acetylcysteine and saline prior to radiocontrast; no benefit of mannitol and diuretics over saline alone
  - Avoid potential nephrotoxic insults such as hypotension, hypovolemia, nephrotoxic agents
  - Maintain adequate renal perfusion
  - Nutritional support recommended but benefit not proven
  - Hemodialysis with intensive protocols including earlier initiation, increased frequency appears to result in improved outcome
  - During recovery phase, monitor electrolytes and volume status closely with post–ATN diuresis

- **Pearl**

Recovery of renal function occurs more often with nonoliguric acute tubular necrosis than when oliguric. The use of diuretics to convert oliguric ATN into the nonoliguric variety, however, does not improve overall prognosis.

Reference

Esson ML et al: Diagnosis and treatment of acute tubular necrosis. Ann Intern Med 2002;137:744. [PMID: 12416948]

Glomerulonephritis, Acute

- **Essentials of Diagnosis**
  - Oliguria, hypertension, edema (especially periorbital distribution), pulmonary congestion, fatigue
  - Nausea, dyspnea, lethargy, pericarditis, encephalopathy if severe renal failure present
  - "Nephritic" urinary sediment with red cell casts, red cells (may be dysmorphic [acanthocytes]), low urinary MCV ([urine/blood MCV < 1]), white cells; variable proteinuria
  - History and physical may identify temporally associated infections or systemic vasculitis
  - Obtain immunological markers: antinuclear antibodies (ANA), antineutrophil cytoplasmic antibodies (ANCA), anti-GBM antibodies, antistreptolysin O (ASO) titer, HIV, hepatitis B/C antibodies, complement, cryoglobulins

- **Differential Diagnosis**
  - IgA nephropathy/Berger disease
  - Henoch-Schönlein purpura
  - Lupus nephritis
  - Goodpasture syndrome and anti-GBM disease
  - Wegener granulomatosis
  - Microscopic polyangiitis and other vasculitides
  - Poststreptococcal GN
  - Hepatitis B and C associated GN
  - Infective endocarditis

- **Treatment**
  - Renal biopsy for pathological confirmation
  - Supportive management with sodium and fluid restriction
  - Blood pressure control
  - Most etiologies require aggressive immunosuppressive regimens such as high-dose steroids and cyclophosphamide
  - Plasmapheresis may be effective in anti-GBM or cryoglobulin-associated diseases
  - Dialysis in renal failure

- **Pearl**

Rapidly progressive glomerulonephritis (RPGN) is associated with a rapid decline in renal function leading to end-stage renal failure within days to weeks. Crescent formation within glomeruli on renal biopsy is the pathological hallmark of this syndrome.

Reference

Vinen CS et al: Acute glomerulonephritis. Postgrad Med J 2003;79:206. [PMID: 12743337]

Hepatorenal Syndrome

- ■ Essentials of Diagnosis
  - • Acute renal failure in conjunction with preexisting liver dysfunction: advanced cirrhosis, severe alcoholic hepatitis, fulminant liver failure
  - • Hyperbilirubinemia, coagulopathy, encephalopathy
  - • Often with stigmata of portal hypertension: varices, ascites
  - • Absence of shock, bacterial infection, nephrotoxic agents
  - • Reduced urine output but rarely anuric
  - • Reduced urinary sodium excretion with $FE_{Na} < 1\%$
  - • Unresponsive to fluid challenge or withdrawal of diuretics
  - • Due to severe vasoconstriction of renal arteries accompanied by extrarenal arterial vasodilation, hypotension
  - • Precipitated by gastrointestinal bleed, spontaneous bacterial peritonitis (SBP), excessive diuresis

- ■ Differential Diagnosis
  - • Volume depletion: diuretics, bleeding
  - • Cardiac pump failure
  - • Obstructive uropathy
  - • Acute tubular necrosis: sepsis, prolonged hypoperfusion
  - • Drug toxicity: NSAIDs, aminoglycosides, contrast
  - • Autoimmune glomerulonephritis: vasculitis, cryoglobulinemia

- ■ Treatment
  - • Restore volume with albumin or blood to euvolemic state
  - • Treat infection including SBP
  - • Splanchnic vasoconstrictors have some reported success: vasopressin, norepinephrine, midodrine combined with octreotide
  - • Peritoneal jugular shunt (LeVeen) benefits not well established; transjugular intrahepatic portosystemic shunt (TIPS) with some anecdotal benefit
  - • Hemodialysis and ultrafiltration
  - • Prevention: avoid nephrotoxins, excess diuresis, large-volume paracentesis
  - • Administration of albumin and antibiotics reduces likelihood renal impairment in setting of SBP

- ■ Pearl

Renal failure in HRS is "functional"; kidneys transplanted from patients with HRS may resume normal function in the recipient, and renal function returns to normal when patients with HRS undergo liver transplantation.

Reference

Kramer L et al: Hepatorenal syndrome. Semin Nephrol 2002;22:290. [PMID: 12118394]

Interstitial Nephritis, Acute

- **Essentials of Diagnosis**
  - Acute decline in renal function with active urinary sediment (not indicative of acute glomerular process)
  - May have history of drug hypersensitivity and associated fever, rash, flank pain
  - Hypertension and edema uncommon
  - Hematuria, sterile pyuria, proteinuria, white cell casts
  - Eosinophiluria often described; but also seen in atheroembolic renal disease, transplant rejection, urinary tract infections
  - FE_{Na} usually >1%
  - May have renal tubular acidosis: proximal or distal
  - Positive gallium scan with prolonged renal uptake (>72 hours) supports diagnosis of allergic interstitial nephritis
  - Pathologically marked interstitial inflammation and edema
  - Overall favorable prognosis; generally reversible

- **Differential Diagnosis**
  - Antibiotics: penicillins, cephalosporins, sulfonamides, rifampin
  - Nonsteroidal anti-inflammatory drugs
  - Diuretics: thiazides, furosemide
  - Infections: streptococcal infections, diphtheria, leptospirosis
  - Acute urate nephropathy, tumor lysis syndrome
  - Ethylene glycol ingestion with calcium oxalate deposition
  - Immunologic disorders: systemic lupus erythematosis (SLE), Sjögren syndrome, mixed essential cryoglobulinemia
  - Acute allograft rejection

- **Treatment**
  - Identify and eliminate possible inciting factors: drugs, infection
  - Steroid use controversial; most often used in drug-induced interstitial nephritis or if renal failure severe, prolonged
  - Pretreatment with allopurinol and forced alkaline diuresis in anticipation of aggressive chemotherapy to decrease risk of urate nephropathy
  - Dialysis may be indicated on temporary or permanent basis

- **Pearl**

The classic triad of fever, rash, and eosinophilia in the setting of acute renal failure is present only in one third of patients with drug-induced allergic interstitial nephritis.

Reference

Kodner CM et al: Diagnosis and management of acute interstitial nephritis. Am Fam Physician 2003;67:2527. [PMID: 12825841]

Pigment Nephropathy: Rhabdomyolysis & Hemolysis

- **Essentials of Diagnosis**
  - Acute renal failure in setting of severe muscle breakdown or hemolysis
  - Dark-colored brown or red urine
  - Muscle pain, weakness may be present in rhabdomyolysis
  - Symptoms of anemia observed in severe hemolysis
  - In rhabdomyolysis: elevated creatinine kinase and aldolase, reduced BUN:creatinine ratio; urine dipstick positive for heme in absence of red cells
  - In hemolysis: elevated serum free hemoglobin, reduced haptoglobin
  - AST and LDH often elevated in both
  - Massive cellular release of myoglobin or hemoglobin toxic to renal tubules
  - Risk factors for pigment nephropathy: reduced renal perfusion states, hypovolemia

- **Differential Diagnosis**
  - Rhabdomyolysis
  - Trauma: crush injury, electric burn, heat stress
  - Excessive contraction: seizure, tetanus, malignant hyperthermia, neuroleptic malignant syndrome
  - Electrolytes: hypokalemia, hypophosphatemia
  - Infection: clostridial toxin (gas gangrene), pyomyositis
  - Polymyositis, dermatomyositis
  - Drugs: combined HMG-CoA reductase inhibitors and fibric acid derivatives, amphetamine
  - Hemolysis: transfusion reactions; drugs and toxins (quinine, fava beans, snake venom); mechanical lysis (prosthetic heart valves, extracorporeal circulation)

- **Treatment**
  - Fluid resuscitation to restore adequate renal perfusion
  - Initiate diuresis with mannitol or furosemide once euvolemic
  - Alkalinization of urine confers theoretical benefits
  - Monitor electrolyte imbalance: hyperkalemia, hypocalcemia, hyperphosphatemia
  - Manage as acute renal failure/acute tubular necrosis

- **Pearl**

In crush injury, especially involving the thighs, patient must be monitored for not only the development of renal failure from rhabdomyolysis but also for compartment syndrome.

Reference

Holt SG: Pathogenesis and treatment of renal dysfunction in rhabdomyolysis. Intensive Care Med 2001;27:803. [PMID: 11430535]

Pulmonary-Renal Syndromes

- **Essentials of Diagnosis**
  - Vasculitic syndromes that involve both lungs and kidneys
  - Cough, dyspnea, hemoptysis, alveolar hemorrhage; may have rash, upper respiratory tract involvement depending on disorder
  - Microscopic hematuria often precedes fulminant renal failure
  - Radiographically diffuse alveolar infiltrates; occasionally cavitary lesions
  - Bronchoalveolar lavage with >20% hemosiderin-laden macrophages indicates alveolar hemorrhage; nonspecific
  - Need to exclude correlated pulmonary and renal disorders: CHF with excessive diuresis, renal failure complicated by pulmonary edema, disseminated infection
  - Drug/toxin exposure history helpful: penicillamine in Goodpasture syndrome, SLE; leukotriene inhibitors in Churg-Strauss syndrome; hydrocarbon in Goodpasture disease; hydralazine, procainamide, quinidine in SLE
  - Serological markers: ANCA, anti-GBM, ANA, anti-dsDNA
  - Definitive diagnosis often with renal biopsy with immunofluorescent staining

- **Differential Diagnosis**
  - Wegener granulomatosis
  - Microscopic polyangiitis
  - Systemic lupus erythematosus (SLE)
  - Goodpasture syndrome
  - Churg-Strauss syndrome

- **Treatment**
  - Maintain adequate airway in massive hemoptysis
  - Hemodialysis may be indicated in acute renal failure
  - Immunosuppressive agents: corticosteroids, cyclophosphamide
  - Plasmapheresis in Goodpasture syndrome
  - Adjunctive trimethoprim-sulfamethoxazole may be considered in Wegener granulomatosis
  - Renal histopathology in SLE often determines treatment

- **Pearl**

Though first believed that leukotriene inhibitors can trigger development of Churg-Strauss syndrome, it is more likely that the use of these medications in steroid-dependent asthmatics unmasks clinical manifestations of a previously suppressed eosinophilic syndrome.

Reference

Rodriguez W et al: Pulmonary-renal syndromes in the intensive care unit. Crit Care Clin 2002;18:881. [PMID: 12418445]

Renal Failure, Acute

- **Essentials of Diagnosis**
  - Abrupt reduction in renal function resulting in azotemia
  - Reduced urine output but may be non-oliguric, anorexia, nausea, vomiting, hiccupping
  - Irritability, asterixis, headache, lethargy, confusion, uremic encephalopathy, coma
  - If pre-renal, orthostatic blood pressure and heart rate; if volume overloaded, jugular venous distension, gallops, rales
  - Pericardial rub, Kussmaul respirations may be seen
  - Hyperkalemia and acidosis can induce cardiac arrhythmias
  - Elevated blood urea nitrogen (BUN) and creatinine (Cr); BUN/Cr > 20 in prerenal azotemia, some obstructive uropathy
  - Fe_{Na} = [(urine Na $\times$ serum Cr)/(urine Cr $\times$ serum Na)] $\times$ 100; <1% in prerenal azotemia; >1% in ATN
  - Urinalysis: pyuria, crystals, stones, hemoglobin, protein, casts, bacteria

- **Differential Diagnosis**
  - Prerenal azotemia: volume depletion, reduced cardiac output, hypotension, renovascular obstruction, NSAIDs, ACE inhibitors
  - Intrinsic renal failure: acute tubular necrosis (ATN), acute glomerulonephritis, acute interstitial nephritis
  - Postrenal azotemia: prostate enlargement, tumor, blood clots, stones, crystals, retroperitoneal fibrosis
  - Hepatorenal syndrome

- **Treatment**
  - Fluid challenge should be considered
  - Avoid nephrotoxic agents: aminoglycosides, NSAIDs, contrast
  - Dietary restriction of sodium, potassium, phosphate, protein
  - Adjust dose of medications that are renally cleared
  - Renal ultrasound useful in evaluating for obstructive process; relieving obstruction essential once identified
  - Renal biopsy indicated if diagnosis elusive or when histological diagnosis important for therapy
  - Dialysis for hyperkalemia, acidosis, fluid overload, uremic symptoms, very catabolic patients (rapid sustained rise in BUN)

- **Pearl**

In complete renal shutdown, the serum creatinine typically increases by 1–2 mg/dL per day. When a more rapid rise is observed, rhabdomyolysis should be considered.

Reference

Abernethy VE et al: Acute renal failure in the critically ill patient. Crit Care Clin 2002;18:203. [PMID: 12053831]

Renal Failure, Drug Clearance in

■ Essential Concepts

- Clearance is rate of drug elimination from body; reduced clearance rates lead to increased drug half-life and potential toxicity
- Renal failure leads to decreased clearance of drugs eliminated by the kidneys
- Dose adjustment important when drugs predominantly renally eliminated; common medications include most antimicrobials, H-2 blocker, low molecular weight heparin, nitroprusside; doses can be adjusted by reducing dose, frequency, or both
- Metabolites of drugs may remain pharmacologically active and accumulate in setting of renal failure: meperidine, procainamide
- Most polypeptides metabolized by kidneys: insulin
- Renal failure may affect liver metabolism: increased liver clearance of nafcillin in end-stage renal disease
- Drug levels can be monitored but interpretation should consider clinical context: aminoglycosides, vancomycin, digoxin, anticonvulsants, theophylline
- Degree of drug removal by dialysis determines need for supplemental dosing

■ Essentials of Management

- Estimate renal function and glomerular filtration rate (GFR) with creatinine clearance (Cl_{cr}) = $[(140\text{-age}) \times (IBW \text{ in kg})]/(72 \times Cr)$, where IBW is ideal body weight
- Monitor rapidity of change in renal function
- Reassess appropriateness of all medication doses and adjust accordingly when renal function changes
- Avoid exclusively relying on nomograms due to complexity and variability of various interactions
- Assess whether drug metabolites pharmacologically active and whether they accumulate in renal failure
- Further modification of drug dosing required when dialysis initiated and depends on mode, frequency and efficiency

■ Pearl

In addition to impaired drug elimination, several other factors pertaining to drug therapy in patients with renal insufficiency are also affected, including drug absorption and volume of distribution.

Reference

Pichette V et al: Drug metabolism in chronic renal failure. Curr Drug Metab 2003;4:91. [PMID: 12678690]

Renal Failure, Prevention

- **Essential Concepts**
  - Acute renal insufficiency associated with increased ICU mortality, but limited studies on renal failure prevention
  - Limited data available in certain settings: cardiovascular surgery, sepsis, contrast-induced nephropathy, cirrhosis associated renal dysfunction
  - Acute tubular necrosis (ATN) and prerenal azotemia most common causes of renal impairment
  - Use of nephrotoxic agents sometimes unavoidable: amphotericin, aminoglycosides, radiographic contrast
  - Clinical use of renal dose dopamine and diuretics of unproven benefit
  - Albumin infusion costly and has limited role
  - Atrial natriuretic peptide restricted to clinical trials

- **Essentials of Management**
  - Avoid use of nephrotoxic agents, if possible
  - Minimize toxicity exposure: once-daily aminoglycoside dosing, liposomal amphotericin B infusions, nonionic contrast agents
  - Maintain adequate renal perfusion with volume expansion; colloid versus crystalloid replacement remains controversial
  - Avoid diuretics unless volume overloaded; exception may be mannitol use in myoglobinuria after volume resuscitation
  - Premedication with N-acetylcysteine protects from contrast nephropathy; fenoldopam also appears to reduce this nephropathy
  - Albumin in conjunction with antibiotics reduced renal impairment and mortality in cirrhosis associated spontaneous bacterial peritonitis
  - Splanchnic vasoconstrictors and TIPS have led to some reversal of hepatorenal syndrome although mortality remains high
  - Selenium replacement promising in sepsis

- **Pearl**

In the face of life-threatening hypoxemia secondary to pulmonary edema, aggressive diuresis takes precedence even in the setting of worsening renal function, as the availability of renal replacement therapies makes "sacrificing" the kidneys an acceptable therapeutic option.

Reference

Block CA et al: Prevention of acute renal failure in the critically ill. Am J Respir Crit Care Med 2002;165:320. [PMID: 11818313]

Renal Replacement Therapy (Hemodialysis)

- **Essential Concepts**
  - Indicated for chronic renal failure with acute illness; acute renal failure unresponsive to other therapy; specific indications with no alternative treatment
  - May be needed emergently for volume overload, uremic complications, hyperkalemia, hypercalcemia, metabolic acidosis; overdose of dialyzable drug
  - Hemodialysis uses semipermeable membrane to separate blood from dialysate fluid; unwanted solutes move into dialysate by diffusion
  - Hemofiltration uses same membrane, solute and water move by convection (high to low pressure); low efficiency of removal of uremic toxins; provide replacement for lost solute and water for desired fluid balance or correction of metabolic acidosis
  - Intermittent hemodialysis (±hemofiltration) 3–7 times/wk, 1–4 hours per session; rapid fluid removal; high blood flow (300 ml/min) may cause hypotension; requires anticoagulation
  - Continuous venovenous hemofiltration and dialysis (CVVHD); blood flow 100 mL/min; usually less hypotension, low constant fluid removal, better tolerated by critically ill patients
  - Acute peritoneal dialysis rarely used in ICU

- **Essentials of Management**
  - Insert venous double-lumen hemodialysis catheter
  - Specify net fluid balance, electrolytes in dialysate, systemic heparin or regional citrate anticoagulation, blood flow, volume of replacement fluids
  - Observe heart rate, blood pressure; monitor for bleeding; record fluid balance; adjust drug dosages to meet increased clearance
  - Complications: infection, bleeding, deep venous thrombosis, hypotension, thrombocytopenia, acid-base and electrolyte disturbances, hypoxemia, arrhythmias, dialysis disequilibrium syndrome

- **Pearl**

When adjusting medications, keep in mind that hemodialysis and CVVHD may have different rates of elimination for different drugs.

Reference

Abdeen O et al: Dialysis modalities in the intensive care unit. Crit Care Clin 2002;18:223. [PMID: 12053832]

15

Rheumatology

Catastrophic Antiphospholipid Syndrome

■ Essentials of Diagnosis
- Multiorgan failure due to systemic small vessel vasoocclusion associated with circulating anticardiolipin antibodies or positive lupus anticoagulant
- Manifestations include: pulmonary insufficiency (ARDS, alveolar hemorrhage, pulmonary infarct); cardiac complications (cardiovascular collapse, valvular lesions, myocardial infarction); CNS abnormalities (altered mental status, seizure); abdominal pain; renal dysfunction; hypertension; livedo reticularis
- Thrombocytopenia and microangiopathic hemolytic anemia
- Risk groups: primary antiphospholipid syndrome (APS) with episodic deep vein thrombosis, thrombocytopenia, or recurrent fetal loss with antiphospholipid antibodies; secondary APS with concomitant SLE
- Precipitating factors: infection, trauma, surgical procedures, withdrawal of anticoagulation therapy

■ Differential Diagnosis
- Disseminated intravascular coagulation (DIC)
- Heparin-induced thrombocytopenia syndrome (HITS)
- Hereditary thrombophilia
- Thrombotic thrombocytopenia purpura (TTP)
- Sepsis syndrome
- Multiple cholesterol emboli

■ Treatment
- Support failing organ systems with mechanical ventilation, vasopressor or inotropic drugs, hemodialysis
- Consider pulmonary artery catheter monitoring to guide fluid resuscitation and pressor support
- Anticoagulation to suppress further thrombosis; higher than usual doses of heparin may be needed
- Corticosteroids to treat possible vasculitis, adrenal insufficiency, reduce cytokine effects
- Other modalities with possible value include fibrinolytic agents, plasmapheresis, cyclophosphamide, intravenous gamma globulin, prostacyclin, danazol, cyclosporine, azathioprine

■ Pearl

Abdominal pain and hypotension in a patient with CAPS may be a sign of adrenal insufficiency in the face of a significant systemic stress.

Reference

Westney GE et al: Catastrophic antiphospholipid syndrome in the intensive care unit. Crit Care Clin 2002;18:805. [PMID: 12418442]

Scleroderma/Progressive Systemic Sclerosis

- ■ Essentials of Diagnosis
  - • Signs and symptoms depend on organ involvement and include dyspnea, fatigue, right-heart failure, cough, hemoptysis, headache, blurred vision
  - • Autoimmune disease characterized by exuberant fibrosis and small-vessel vasculopathy involving skin, lungs, heart, gastrointestinal tract, musculoskeletal system
  - • Two major subsets: limited cutaneous sclerosis (CREST syndrome with calcinosis cutis, Raynaud phenomenon, esophageal dysmotility, sclerodactyly, telangiectasias) with indolent course; diffuse systemic sclerosis with aggressive course
  - • Complications requiring ICU care: pulmonary hypertension, aspiration pneumonia, alveolar hemorrhage, renal crisis with malignant hypertension
  - • Skin involvement may make intravenous access difficult

- ■ Differential Diagnosis
  - • Pulmonary hypertension: primary or drug-induced, valvular heart disease
  - • Aspiration pneumonia: community-acquired pneumonia, acute interstitial pneumonitis
  - • Alveolar hemorrhage: bleeding telangiectasias, ARDS

- ■ Treatment
  - • Treatment targets systemic inflammation with immunosuppressive agents such as prednisone, cyclophosphamide
  - • Hyperalimentation may be required if GI involvement causes malabsorption, malnutrition, pseudoobstruction
  - • Elevate head of bed, prokinetic agents, acid-suppressing drugs to reduce aspiration pneumonia risk
  - • Pulmonary hypertension may benefit from oxygen, pulmonary vasodilators, cardiac inotropic agents, diuretics
  - • Renal crisis: avoid corticosteroids; aggressive blood pressure control; ACE inhibitors for treatment and prophylaxis; hemodialysis for hyperkalemia or uremia

- ■ Pearl

Scleroderma renal crisis, typically characterized by hypertension and a rapidly rising creatinine, has been associated with the antecedent use of high-dose corticosteroids.

Reference

Cossio M et al: Life-threatening complications of systemic sclerosis. Crit Care Clin 2002;18:819. [PMID: 12418443]

Systemic Lupus Erythematosus (SLE)

- **■ Essentials of Diagnosis**
  - Symptoms depend on organ system involved and include dyspnea, hemoptysis, altered mental status, cerebral dysfunction, chest pain, fever
  - Systemic autoimmune disorder that can affect multiple organ systems
  - Complications requiring ICU care: acute lupus pneumonitis, alveolar hemorrhage, lupus cerebritis, seizures, premature atherosclerotic coronary artery disease, pericarditis, myocarditis, bowel perforation, pancreatitis
  - Infection important cause of ICU admission: bacteria account for >90% including *Streptococcus pneumoniae*, *Staphylococcus aureus*, Enterobacteriaceae, nonfermentative gram-negative rods, *Salmonella*
  - Chronic steroid use increases risk of lung and brain infection with *Nocardia*

- **■ Differential Diagnosis**
  - Lung: pleuritis, alveolar hemorrhage, community-acquired pneumonia, ARDS
  - CNS: seizure, stroke, meningitis
  - Cardiovascular: pericarditis, pericardial effusion, myocarditis, myocardial infarction, vasculitis
  - Gastrointestinal: mesenteric thrombosis, ischemic bowel, ruptured hepatic aneurysm, cholecystitis, pancreatitis

- **■ Treatment**
  - Empiric broad-spectrum antibiotics until infection excluded; if routine cultures nonrevealing, bronchoscopy or open-lung biopsy may be necessary if lungs involved
  - Severe noninfectious complications typically treated with corticosteroids
  - Adjunctive immunosuppressive therapy with cyclophosphamide, azathioprine can be considered in conjunction with plasmapheresis in certain patients

- **■ Pearl**

Infections are the leading cause of morbidity and mortality in patients with SLE and can be difficult to discern from an exacerbation of this autoimmune disease.

Reference

Raj R et al: Systemic lupus erythematosus in the intensive care unit. Crit Care Clin 2002;18:781. [PMID: 12418441]

Vasculitis

- **Essentials of Diagnosis**
  - Signs and symptoms overlap with infection, connective tissues diseases, and malignancy; include fever, rash, neuropathy, visual disturbances, upper-airway symptoms, weight loss, malaise, myalgias, arthralgias
  - Vasculitides that may require ICU care: Wegener granulomatosis, microscopic polyangiitis, small-vessel vasculitis associated with antineutrophil cytoplasmic antibodies (ANCA)
  - Causes of deterioration: active vasculitis, complication of medical therapy, overwhelming infection
  - May have anemia, thrombocytopenia, leukocytosis or leukopenia, elevated BUN and creatinine, active urinary sediment, reduced complement levels, elevated ESR or CRP
  - Leukopenia concerning for drug toxicity or infection
  - Specific serologies to evaluate known or suspected vasculitis include ANA, ANCA, anti-GBM
  - Diagnosis made by combination of characteristic clinical, laboratory, radiologic, pathologic features; biopsy of involved organ frequently diagnostic
  - Underlying vasculitis should be suspected in alveolar hemorrhage syndromes, rapidly progressive glomerulonephritis, pulmonary-renal syndromes

- **Differential Diagnosis**
  - Collagen vascular disease   • Endocarditis
  - Malignancy with paraneoplastic syndrome

- **Treatment**
  - Regardless of type and severity of vasculitis, general approach involves immunosuppression with corticosteroids often in conjunction with cyclophosphamide
  - Close attention to medication dosing based on renal function and degree of bone marrow suppression
  - Plasma exchange for severe renal impairment and some forms of diffuse alveolar hemorrhage

- **Pearl**

Distinguishing between a flare-up of the underlying vasculitis from infection or toxicity from medical therapy is extremely important because the therapy for one is contraindicated in the management of the other.

Reference

Frankel SK et al: Vasculitis: Wegener granulomatosis, Churg-Strauss syndrome, microscopic polyangiitis, polyarteritis nodosa, and Takayasu arteritis. Crit Care Clin 2002;18:855. [PMID: 12418444]

16

Toxicology

Acetaminophen Overdose

- **Essentials of Diagnosis**
  - Minimal symptoms in first 24 hours; possible nausea, vomiting, diaphoresis, and lethargy
  - 24–48 hours postingestion, onset of hepatic AST, ALT elevation
  - 3–4 days postingestion: progressive hepatic damage, nausea, vomiting, jaundice, right upper-quadrant pain, asterixis, bleeding, lethargy, coma
  - In adults, <125 mg/kg rarely produce toxicity; 125–250 mg/kg variably cause toxicity; doses >250 mg/kg high risk for liver failure; patients with liver disease more susceptible to toxicity
  - Acetaminophen-containing combination medications should be considered in all overdose patients

- **Differential Diagnosis**
  - Severe viral or alcoholic hepatitis
  - Cyclopeptide toxicity from mushroom ingestion

- **Treatment**
  - Acetaminophen level >4 hours postingestion >150 μg/mL toxic; use nomogram to ascertain risk for other time points
  - Gastric lavage if within 2–4 hours of ingestion
  - Give N-acetylcysteine to patients with suspected or known ingestion of toxic dose or who have toxic levels by nomogram; most effective if given within 8 hours of ingestion
  - N-acetylcysteine dose 140 mg/kg orally followed by 70 mg/kg orally every 4 hours for 17 doses
  - Intravenous N-acetylcysteine can be given (not approved in US) if cannot tolerate oral
  - Supportive care for consequences of hepatic failure: vitamin K for coagulopathy, lactulose for encephalopathy
  - Liver transplantation should be considered in appropriate patients who are refractory to treatment

- **Pearl**

Laboratories may use different units for acetaminophen level, as it can be reported in μg/mL (toxic >150 μg/mL at 4 h), μmol/L (toxic >1000 μmol/L at 4 h), or mg% (15 mg% = 150 μg/mL).

Reference

Mokhlesi B et al: Adult toxicology in critical care: Part II: specific poisonings. Chest 2003;123:897. [PMID: 12628894]

Alcohol Withdrawal

■ **Essentials of Diagnosis**

- Generalized coarse tremors starting 6–8 hours after last drink, intensifying up to 24–36 hours
- Anxiety, insomnia, anorexia, sweating, facial flushing, mydriasis, tachycardia, and hypertension seen in first days; altered mental status, nightmares, auditory hallucinations in 25% of patients, peaking 24–36 hours
- Generalized tonic-clonic seizures in one third of patients, usually within 12–24 hours; status epilepticus in 3%; patients with previous alcohol withdrawal seizures more likely to have recurrent seizures
- Delirium tremens in 5%, 2–4 days after last drink; confusion, insomnia, vivid hallucinations, delusions, tremor, mydriasis, tachycardia, fever, diaphoresis; may last 1–3 days and relapse over weeks

■ **Differential Diagnosis**

- Hypoglycemia
- Anticholinergic or stimulant overdose
- Sedative withdrawal
- CNS infection, sepsis, thyrotoxicosis

■ **Treatment**

- Supportive care, including IV fluids as needed
- Thiamine 100 mg intravenously, folate, multivitamins
- Benzodiazepines for withdrawal symptoms on an as-needed basis, rather than scheduled dosing
- Benzodiazepines for seizures
- For delirium tremens, aggressive intravenous hydration, may require high-dose benzodiazepines, such as diazepam 5–10 mg intravenously every 1–4 hours

■ **Pearl**

Watch for the presence of other behavioral health problems such as depression in alcoholic patients.

Reference

Korsten TR, O'Connor PG: Management of drug and alcohol withdrawal. N Engl J Med 2003;348:1786. [PMID: 12724485]

Benzodiazepine Withdrawal

- ■ Essentials of Diagnosis
  - Anxiety, irritability, dysphoria, insomnia, confusion, disorientation; may have hypertension, tachycardia, diaphoresis, tremors, hyperthermia, seizures
  - May be due to complete benzodiazepine abstinence, reduced intake, or administration of GABA receptor antagonist such as flumazenil
  - Timing of symptom onset depends on half-life of medication being chronically taken by the patient; <24 hours after withdrawal from alprazolam, >1 week after withdrawal from diazepam
  - Symptoms of withdrawal similar to ethanol withdrawal

- ■ Differential Diagnosis
  - Ethanol withdrawal
  - Hypoglycemia
  - Anticholinergic or stimulant overdose
  - CNS infection, sepsis, thyrotoxicosis

- ■ Treatment
  - Supportive care, including IV fluids as needed
  - Stabilize withdrawal symptoms by administration of long-acting benzodiazepine such as diazepam; once stabilized, withdraw long-acting benzodiazepine dose by about 10% per day
  - IV diazepam for seizures
  - If withdrawal precipitated by flumazenil, supportive care will usually suffice, as half-life of flumazenil is very short

- ■ Pearl

More than 10% of adults in the United States use benzodiazepines on a regular basis.

Reference

Jenkins DH: Substance abuse and withdrawal in the intensive care unit. Contemporary issues. Surg Clin North Am 2000;80:1033. [PMID: 10897277]

Beta-Adrenergic Blocker Overdose

- **Essentials of Diagnosis**
  - Hypotension, bradycardia, heart block
  - Can also cause altered mental status, hallucinations, seizures, hypoglycemia
  - In severe overdose, may have cardiogenic shock

- **Differential Diagnosis**
  - Calcium channel blocker overdose
  - Barbiturate overdose
  - Antiarrhythmic toxicity
  - Tricyclic antidepressant toxicity

- **Treatment**
  - Supportive care
  - Gastric lavage for patients within 2–4 hours of ingestion; activated charcoal and cathartic agents
  - Glucagon is most effective agent for reversing bradycardia and hypotension; typical dose 0.05 mg/kg intravenously followed by infusion of 0.07 mg/kg/h as needed
  - Atropine for symptomatic bradycardia; consider dopamine or norepinephrine
  - If refractory to therapy, consider cardiac pacemaker, isoproterenol, intra-aortic balloon pump
  - Charcoal hemoperfusion may be useful for atenolol or nadolol, which have small volume of distribution with limited protein binding

- **Pearl**

Side effects of glucagon include nausea, vomiting, hyperglycemia, hypokalemia, and allergic reactions.

Reference

Kerns W II et al: Beta-blocker and calcium channel blocker toxicity. Emerg Med Clin North Am 1994;12:365. [PMID: 7910555]

Calcium Channel Blocker Overdose

- ■ Essentials of Diagnosis
  - • Bradycardia, hypotension, heart block, and asystole
  - • Drowsiness, metabolic acidosis, hyperglycemia, seizure, and coma may also be seen

- ■ Differential Diagnosis
  - • Beta-blocker toxicity
  - • Barbiturate overdose
  - • Antiarrhythmic toxicity
  - • Tricyclic antidepressant toxicity

- ■ Treatment
  - • Supportive care
  - • Gastric lavage for patients within 2–4 hours of ingestion; activated charcoal and cathartic agents if acute ingestion
  - • For cardiotoxicity: calcium chloride, 10% 10 mL intravenously, or calcium gluconate, 30 mL intravenously initially, followed by repeated doses if needed
  - • Glucagon, 0.1 mg/kg intravenous bolus followed by 0.1 mg/kg/h drip, if intravenous calcium ineffective
  - • Atropine and vasopressor agents such as dopamine or dobutamine in patients refractory to treatment

- ■ Pearl

Large ingestions of sustained-release preparations may result in formation of stomach concretions. Whole-bowel irrigation has been suggested for use in such ingestions.

Reference

Proano L et al: Calcium channel blocker overdose. Am J Emerg Med 1995;13:444. [PMID: 7605536]

Cocaine

- **Essentials of Diagnosis**
  - Tachycardia, hypertension, hyperthermia, agitation, and seizures
  - Cardiac dysrhythmias, including atrial fibrillation or tachycardia, ventricular tachycardia, or asystole
  - End-organ ischemia can cause stroke, myocardial infarction, bowel ischemia, renal infarction, limb ischemia; severe hypertension can lead to intracranial hemorrhage (subarachnoid or intraparenchymal) or aortic dissection
  - Pneumothorax or pneumomediastinum can be seen when cocaine smoked or snorted
  - Excess muscle activity can lead to rhabdomyolysis or hyperthermia
  - Can be used by snorting, smoking, or intravenous injection

- **Differential Diagnosis**
  - Sympathomimetic, theophylline, phencyclidine intoxication
  - Ethanol or benzodiazepine withdrawal
  - Thyrotoxicosis
  - CNS infection

- **Treatment**
  - Supportive care
  - Active cooling measures for hyperthermia
  - Benzodiazepines for agitation and seizures
  - Phenobarbital or phenytoin for seizures refractory to benzodiazepines
  - Intravenous nitroprusside for severe hypertension
  - If myocardial ischemia or infarction, usual therapy except avoid beta blockers because of potential for severe hypertension from unopposed alpha-adrenergic stimulation; phentolamine may be used for coronary vasospasm
  - Intravenous fluids and alkalinization of urine for rhabdomyolysis

- **Pearl**

Lidocaine is often ineffective for cocaine-induced ventricular dysrhythmias; consider cocaine toxicity in a young otherwise healthy patient in an agitated state with ventricular dysrhythmia unresponsive to lidocaine.

Reference

Shanti CM, Lucas CE: Cocaine and the critical care challenge. Crit Care Med 2003;31:1851. [PMID: 12794430]

Digitalis Toxicity

- **Essentials of Diagnosis**
  - Most asymptomatic but may have anorexia, nausea, vomiting, visual changes (amblyopia, photophobia, scotomata, yellow halos), abdominal pain, headache, hallucinations, drowsiness
  - Cardiac dysrhythmias of virtually any type can occur, including bradycardia, AV dissociation, supraventricular tachycardia, ventricular tachyarrhythmias
  - Toxicity can occur from acute, chronic, or acute plus chronic use; potential for toxicity increased by age, coexisting conditions, hypokalemia, hypomagnesemia, hypercalcemia, hypoxia, other cardiac medications
  - High potassium and digoxin levels seen in acute, but not necessarily with chronic toxicity

- **Differential Diagnosis**
  - Ingestion of cardiac glycoside-containing plants, including foxglove, oleander, lily of the valley, dogbane, red squill
  - Calcium channel blocker, beta-adrenergic blockers
  - Tricyclic antidepressant overdose

- **Treatment**
  - Discontinue digitalis
  - Emesis or gastric lavage if recent ingestion; multidose activated charcoal may be beneficial even if substantial time elapsed from ingestion due to enterohepatic recirculation
  - Monitor cardiac rhythm
  - Check electrolytes, digitalis level; replace potassium and magnesium if low
  - Purified digoxin-specific antibodies (Fab) indicated for ventricular arrhythmias, bradyarrhythmias, severe hyperkalemia with potassium level >5.0 mEq/L, or digoxin level exceeding 10–15 ng/mL
  - If digoxin-specific Fab not available in face of ventricular arrhythmia, phenytoin and lidocaine are drugs of choice

- **Pearl**

Hyperkalemia from digitalis toxicity should not be treated with intravenous calcium chloride, as this may exacerbate intracellular hypercalcemia and cause intractable ventricular tachyarrhythmias.

Reference

Eichhorn EJ, Gheorghiade M: Digoxin. Prog Cardiovasc Dis 2002;44:251. [PMID: 12007081]

Iron Overdose

- ## Essentials of Diagnosis
  - GI symptoms <2 hours; abdominal pain, vomiting, diarrhea, hematemesis, hematochezia; few symptoms seen 6–24 hours postingestion
  - Shock, coma, coagulopathy, acidosis, multisystem organ failure may occur after 6–72 hours; most deaths occur during this phase
  - Hepatic necrosis occurs within 48 hours of ingestion with or without shock; second most common cause of death
  - Late complications: bowel obstruction at 2–4 weeks
  - Iron overdose during pregnancy associated with spontaneous abortion, preterm delivery, maternal death
  - Serum iron level drawn 4–6 hours postingestion >500 μg/dL significant; prognosis worsens with level >1000 μg/dL; levels drawn >6 hours postingestion not useful
  - Iron tablets seen on abdominal radiographs verify ingestion

- ## Differential Diagnosis
  - Other causes of acute abdominal pain or GI bleeding

- ## Treatment
  - Gastric lavage with large-bore tube followed by whole-bowel irrigation, particularly if tablets seen on abdominal radiograph
  - Chelation therapy for severe abdominal symptoms, altered mental status, evidence of systemic hypoperfusion, or serum iron level >500 μg/dL
  - Chelation with intravenous deferoxamine, usually 15 mg/kg/h; stop when symptoms resolved, serum iron level <150 μg/dL, metabolic acidosis gone, urine color returns to normal
  - Deferoxamine should only be given after intravascular volume deficits corrected to avoid acute renal failure; IV deferoxamine administration >24–48 hours may precipitate acute respiratory distress syndrome
  - Evaluation for liver transplantation if acute hepatic necrosis

- ## Pearl

If GI symptoms do not occur within 6 hours of ingestion, iron ingestion was likely nontoxic unless the patient ingested enteric-coated iron.

Reference

Tran T et al: Intentional iron overdose in pregnancy—management and outcome. J Emerg Med 2000;18:225. [PMID: 10699527]

Ketamine & Phencyclidine (PCP)

- ■ Essentials of Diagnosis
  - • Ketamine: short-acting anesthetic; no respiratory or cardiovascular depression, but hallucinations; analog of phencyclidine (PCP); both abused as hallucinogens
  - • PCP usage declining, recently increasing ketamine abuse
  - • Variable symptoms and signs; euphoria, agitation, psychosis, violent behavior, seizures; fully alert to comatose
  - • Nystagmus (horizontal, vertical, rotatory) >50% of PCP (rare with ketamine); hypertension, tachycardia
  - • Ketamine inhaled or injected; effects rare >1 hour; PCP smoked, intranasal, or ingested; rapidly absorbed; half-life 7–72 hours
  - • Complicated by rhabdomyolysis, renal failure, concealed injuries due to violent behavior
  - • Urine PCP level confirms diagnosis; serum creatine kinase levels, urine myoglobin

- ■ Differential Diagnosis
  - • Sympathomimetics
  - • Long-acting hallucinogens (3,4-methylenedioxymethamphetamine ("ecstasy"), LSD
  - • Sedative-hypnotics, alcohol; withdrawal from these
  - • Head trauma, meningitis, encephalitis
  - • Psychiatric disorders
  - • Metabolic derangements

- ■ Treatment
  - • Ketamine generally none; rapid elimination
  - • PCP: gastric lavage if suspected large ingestion within 1 hour or co-ingestion suspected; follow with multidose activated charcoal
  - • Supportive care for hypertension, tachycardia; treat hyperthermia
  - • Treat seizures with benzodiazepines, phenytoin
  - • IV fluids, mannitol, bicarbonate for rhabdomyolysis to reduce risk of renal failure
  - • Avoid excessive stimulation; use benzodiazepines or haloperidol for sedation

- ■ Pearl

Some patients suspected of head trauma instead have PCP intoxication.

Reference

Weiner AL et al: Ketamine abusers presenting to the emergency department: a case series. J Emerg Med 2000;18:447. [PMID: 10802423]

Lithium

- **Essentials of Diagnosis**
  - May be acute, chronic, or acute plus chronic lithium toxicity
  - CNS symptoms include tremor, weakness, hyperreflexia, muscle rigidity, slurred speech, tinnitus, seizures, confusion, coma; GI symptoms more common with acute toxicity, including nausea and vomiting
  - May have prolonged QT interval, ST and T wave abnormalities, myocarditis, cardiovascular collapse (rare)
  - Nephrogenic diabetes insipidus in 20–70%
  - Thyrotoxicosis, hyperthermia, hyperparathyroidism, hypercalcemia
  - Risk factors for toxicity in patients previously stable on lithium therapy include ACE inhibitors, NSAIDs, loop diuretics, thiazides, volume depletion, decreased sodium intake, renal insufficiency
  - Serum lithium level >1.5 mEq/L is toxic

- **Differential Diagnosis**
  - Stroke, meningitis, tardive dyskinesia, other CNS disorders
  - Neuroleptic malignant syndrome
  - Sedative-hypnotic or ethanol withdrawal
  - Psychotropic or stimulant overdose

- **Treatment**
  - Gastric lavage, with whole bowel irrigation for significant ingestions
  - Maintenance of fluid and electrolyte balance
  - Hemodialysis effective; should be considered early in ingestion of sustained-release preparations, chronic ingestions with toxicity, with impaired renal function, if neurologic findings, or if serum lithium >4.0 mEq/L

- **Pearl**

As lithium is not metabolized and is eliminated entirely via the kidney, any patient with abnormal renal function should be considered a hemodialysis candidate if there are signs of toxicity.

Reference

Timmer RT, Sands JM: Lithium intoxication. J Am Soc Nephrol 1999;10:666. [PMID: 10073618]

Methanol, Ethylene Glycol, & Isopropanol

■ Essentials of Diagnosis

- Methanol: 12–24 hours after ingestion, visual disturbances, headache, nausea, vomiting, abdominal pain, lethargy, confusion, seizures, coma; retinal and optic disc abnormalities; methanol found in solvents, paint thinners
- Ethylene glycol: First 12 hours, CNS abnormalities; 12–24 hours after ingestion, cardiopulmonary abnormalities including hypertension, high-output cardiac failure, tachycardia; 24–72 hours after ingestion see renal failure, flank pain; may have oxalate crystalluria; ethylene glycol found in antifreeze
- Isopropanol: headache, dizziness, confusion, abdominal pain, nausea, vomiting; isopropanol found in rubbing alcohol, skin and hair products
- Prior to metabolism, all produce increased osmolal gap; all metabolized by alcohol dehydrogenase to toxic metabolites: methanol to formic acid, ethylene glycol to oxalic acid, and isopropanol to acetone; therefore, methanol and ethylene glycol, but not isopropanol, have increased anion gap

■ Differential Diagnosis

- Ethanol intoxication
- Sepsis, meningitis
- Hyperglycemia
- Other causes of anion gap acidosis

■ Treatment

- Supportive care, including IV fluids, oxygen, monitoring
- Gastric decontamination if within 2 hours
- Bicarbonate for severe acidosis with methanol and ethylene glycol
- Folic acid 50 mg intravenously every 4 hours for methanol; thiamine, pyridoxine for ethylene glycol ingestion
- Ethanol infusion to achieve blood ethanol level of 100–150 mg/dL for methanol and ethylene glycol toxicity; saturates alcohol dehydrogenase, preventing formation of toxic metabolites
- Fomepizole (4-methylpyrazole), an alcohol dehydrogenase inhibitor, may be used as an alternative to ethanol
- Hemodialysis for severe toxicity

■ Pearl

A large ingestion of any toxic alcohol, including benzyl alcohol, propylene glycol, isopropanol, methanol, or ethylene glycol will cause elevation of serum osmolality.

Reference

Brent J, et al: Fomepizole for the treatment of methanol poisoning. N Engl J Med 2001;344:424. [PMID: 11172179]

Opioid Overdose

- **Essentials of Diagnosis**
  - Depressed level of consciousness, decreased respirations, which can be pronounced, miotic pupils
  - Less commonly pulmonary edema, hypo- or hyperthermia, emesis, hypoxia, hypotension, depressed deep tendon reflexes

- **Differential Diagnosis**
  - Alcohol intoxication
  - Sedative-hypnotic overdose
  - Cardiogenic pulmonary edema
  - Altered mental status due to CNS infection, encephalopathy, hypoglycemia, seizure, hypothyroidism, stroke

- **Treatment**
  - Send blood for electrolytes, toxicology screen, blood gases, liver function tests; ethanol and acetaminophen levels to evaluate for co-ingestion
  - CXR to evaluate for pulmonary edema or aspiration pneumonia
  - Establish airway and ventilation in the comatose patient
  - Patients with respiratory depression should receive naloxone, 2 mg IV initially; may be repeated up to a total of 10–20 mg if no reversal of symptoms follows initial dose
  - Patients with central nervous system depression without respiratory depression should receive naloxone 0.1–0.4 mg IV initially; partial or absent responses should be followed by naloxone 2 mg IV as described for patients with respiratory depression
  - Continuous naloxone infusion or repeated naloxone doses every 20–60 minutes may be required following initial response, especially when long-acting narcotics have been ingested
  - Gastrointestinal decontamination with nasogastric lavage followed by activated charcoal and a cathartic can be helpful

- **Pearl**

Acute complications of narcotic use due to sharing of needles include pulmonary hypertension, endocarditis, necrotizing fasciitis, and tetanus.

Reference

Watson WA et al: Opioid toxicity recurrence after an initial response to naloxone. J Toxicol Clin Toxicol 1998;36:11. [PMID: 9541035]

Opioid Withdrawal

■ Essentials of Diagnosis

- Early symptoms include lacrimation, rhinorrhea, perspiration, yawning; later see restlessness, piloerection, mydriasis, insomnia, nausea, vomiting, abdominal cramps, diarrhea
- Can see hyperthermia and hypertension in severe cases
- Frequently see intense drug craving
- Symptoms develop when opioid stopped or opiate antagonist administered; timing of symptom onset depends on half-life of opioid
- For heroin, onset of withdrawal symptoms 6 hours after last dose, peak withdrawal symptoms 36–48 hours after last dose, resolution of withdrawal by 4–5 days
- For methadone, onset of withdrawal symptoms 2–3 days after last dose, with withdrawal resolution after 2 weeks
- Sudden onset of withdrawal can be precipitated by administration of naloxone to opiate-dependent patients

■ Differential Diagnosis

- Ethanol withdrawal
- Benzodiazepine withdrawal

■ Treatment

- IV fluids, particularly if there is vomiting and diarrhea
- Control withdrawal symptoms with long-acting opioid such as methadone, 10 mg intramuscularly initially, which is often adequate to control withdrawal symptoms; additional doses administered hourly until symptoms subside, usually 20–40 mg
- Clonidine, 0.1–0.2 mg every 6 hours can be used to treat mild opioid withdrawal

■ Pearl

Patients with pure opioid withdrawal maintain normal mental status. Therefore, altered mental status should prompt a search for other factors contributing to the patient's condition.

Reference

Jenkins DH: Substance abuse and withdrawal in the intensive care unit. Contemporary issues. Surg Clin North Am 2000;80:1033. [PMID: 10897277]

Organophosphate Poisoning

- **Essentials of Diagnosis**
  - Peripheral muscarinic effects: salivation, lacrimation, urinary incontinence, diarrhea, (SLUD syndrome); bronchospasm, bronchorrhea, nausea, vomiting, miosis, blurred vision, diaphoresis
  - Peripheral nicotinic effects: muscle fasciculations, weakness, ataxia, paralysis.
  - CNS effects: headache, slurred speech, confusion, seizures, coma, depressed ventilatory drive
  - Death from respiratory center depression, respiratory muscle weakness, bronchospasm, and bronchial secretions
  - Found in insecticides and herbicides; exposure due to dermal exposure or ingestion; inactivation of acetylcholinesterases with excessive stimulation of cholinergic receptors
  - No definitive laboratory test available; diagnosis based on clinical syndrome and response to therapy; cholinesterase activity level can be obtained, but may take days for results

- **Differential Diagnosis**
  - Myasthenia gravis with cholinergic crisis

- **Treatment**
  - Irrigate areas of dermal exposure copiously
  - Gastric lavage if ingestion within one hour, followed by activated charcoal
  - Intubation and ventilatory support should be considered early
  - Atropine to reverse peripheral muscarinic effects; does not reverse skeletal nicotinic effects
  - Atropine for diagnostic testing: 1 mg IV; watch for papillary dilatation and increase in heart rate; if no response, cholinergic toxicity suggested
  - Atropine for treatment: 2–4 mg intravenously every 10–15 minutes until drying of secretions
  - Pralidoxime reverses nicotinic muscle effects; give with atropine in dose of 25–50 mg/kg over 5–15 minutes; observe for increased muscle strength; can repeat every 4–12 hours as needed

- **Pearl**

Chemical weapons known as nerve agents are a very toxic group of organophosphates; these should be considered in a chemical attack.

Reference

Leikin JB et al: A review of nerve agent exposure for the critical care physician. Crit Care Med 2002;30:2346. [PMID: 12394966]

Salicylate Poisoning

- Essentials of Diagnosis
  - Nausea, vomiting, abdominal pain, hematemesis, tinnitus; lethargy, confusion, coma, seizures
  - Noncardiogenic pulmonary edema
  - Hypoglycemia, hyperthermia
  - Cardiovascular collapse
  - Positive urine ferric chloride or Phenistix test confirms salicylate use
  - Arterial blood gases may show respiratory alkalosis with metabolic acidosis
  - Salicylate levels peak 4–6 hours after ingestion, or later with enteric-coated preparations
  - Dose nomogram estimates severity of acute, but not chronic, toxicity

- Differential Diagnosis
  - Stimulant toxicity
  - Meningitis, encephalitis
  - Pneumonia
  - Renal Failure
  - Diabetic or alcoholic ketoacidosis

- Treatment
  - Maintenance of airway with continuation of respiratory alkalosis
  - Gastric lavage for ingestion of greater than 100 mg/kg within 2 hours of ingestion, or later if enteric-coated preparation
  - Activated charcoal and cathartics
  - Fluid and electrolyte replacement
  - Urinary alkalinization for patients with salicylate levels greater than 35 mg/dL, or levels less than 35 mg/dL with significant symptoms
  - Hemodialysis for salicylate level greater than 100 mg/dL, severe fluid and electrolyte abnormalities, persistent CNS disturbances, or hepatic, pulmonary or renal failure

- Pearl

Maintenance of high pH via respiratory alkalosis and urinary alkalinization prevents salicylates from leaving the blood and entering the CNS.

Reference

Dargan PI et al: An evidence based flowchart to guide the management of acute salicylate (aspirin) overdose. Emerg Med J 2002;19:206. [PMID: 11971828]

Sedative-Hypnotic Overdose

- **Essentials of Diagnosis**
  - Altered sensorium, confusion, dysarthria, ataxia, lethargy, stupor; initial symptoms similar to alcohol intoxication
  - With severe overdose, coma, respiratory and cardiovascular collapse
  - Horizontal and vertical nystagmus, depressed deep tendon reflexes, slow shallow respiratory efforts, pulmonary edema
  - All sedative-hypnotics similar except for duration of action, potential for prolonged effects, especially non-barbiturate/non-benzodiazepines, such as chloral hydrate, ethchlorvynol, glutethimide, meprobamate, methaqualone, methyprylon

- **Differential Diagnosis**
  - Uremia
  - Hepatic encephalopathy
  - Hypoglycemia, hypothyroidism
  - Stroke, seizure, CNS infection

- **Treatment**
  - Always have concern about co-ingestions
  - Intubation for airway protection if cough and gag reflexes are depressed; fluid volume resuscitation for hypotension; vasopressors occasionally required for refractory hypotension
  - Gastric lavage if ingestion within previous 45 minutes; multi-dose activated charcoal decreases absorption and enhances elimination in life-threatening phenobarbital overdose
  - Mannitol-induced diuresis and alkalinization aid in excretion of long-acting barbiturates, but not other agents

- **Pearl**

Bromide intoxication can cause abnormalities in anion gap determination because the autoanalyzer cannot distinguish between bromide and chloride. Therefore, patients with altered mental status, high serum chloride, and narrow anion gap should have a bromide level measured.

Reference

Mokhlesi B et al: Adult toxicology in critical care: Part II: specific poisonings. Chest 2003;123:897. [PMID: 12628894]

Sympathomimetic Overdose

- **Essentials of Diagnosis**
  - Confusion, tremor, paranoia, anxiety, agitation and irritability
  - Mydriasis, tachyarrhythmias, hypertension, hyperreflexia, seizures, hyperthermia, rhabdomyolysis, and renal failure
  - Overdose of prescribed drugs (methylphenidate, dextroamphetamine, ephedrine, pseudoephedrine, diethylpropion, phentermine) or use of recreational agents such as methamphetamine ("crank") or 3,4-methylenedioxymethamphetamine ("ecstasy")
  - In severe cases, life-threatening hyperthermia, arrhythmias, status epilepticus, intracranial hemorrhage, aspiration pneumonia, acute hepatic failure

- **Differential Diagnosis**
  - Thyrotoxicosis
  - CNS infection
  - Ethanol or benzodiazepine withdrawal
  - Toxicity from theophylline, tricyclic antidepressants, anticholinergics, isoniazid, phencyclidine, salicylates

- **Treatment**
  - Supportive care, maintenance of airway and mechanical ventilation if needed
  - Gastric lavage within 2 hours of ingestion; activated charcoal and cathartic
  - Active cooling for rectal temperatures >40°C
  - Evaluation of electrolytes and CK
  - Phentolamine or nitroprusside can be used for severe hypertension
  - Beta-adrenergic blockers (esmolol or propranolol) for tachyarrhythmias
  - For severe agitation, benzodiazepines, phenothiazines, or haloperidol
  - Phenobarbital or phenytoin for seizures

- **Pearl**

While duration of toxicity is usually limited for most sympathomimetics, duration may be prolonged if patients have ingested bags containing the drug for illicit transport ("body-packing") or have used "ice," a long-acting smokable form of methamphetamine.

Reference

Mokhlesi B et al:Adult toxicology in critical care: Part II: specific poisonings. Chest 2003;123:897. [PMID: 12628894]

Theophylline Overdose

- **Essentials of Diagnosis**
  - Nausea and vomiting
  - Cardiac: atrial fibrillation, multifocal atrial tachycardia, ventricular tachyarrhythmias; central nervous system: agitation, hyperreflexia, tremors, seizures; hypotension due to peripheral beta-adrenergic stimulation with vasodilation; hypokalemia in acute ingestion may be refractory to replacement
  - Acute intoxications at serum levels 80–100 μg/mL; with chronic toxicity, serious effects as low as 40 μg/mL

- **Differential Diagnosis**
  - Tricyclic antidepressant, anticholinergic, phenothiazine, caffeine overdose
  - Meningitis, sepsis   • Alcohol withdrawal

- **Treatment**
  - Gastric lavage within 1 hour of ingestion, or within 3–4 hours if sustained-release form ingested
  - Activated charcoal essential; administer 1–2 g/kg regardless of time since ingestion, then 0.5–1 g/kg every 2 hours; do not give cathartics after first dose
  - IV fluids for hypotension; follow with alpha-adrenergic agonists such as phenylephrine, if necessary; beta-adrenergic blockers may be helpful to reverse peripheral beta-adrenergic mediated vasodilatation
  - Verapamil or beta blockers for supraventricular arrhythmias; correct hypokalemia and lidocaine for ventricular dysrhythmias
  - Benzodiazepines, dilantin, or phenobarbital for seizures
  - Hemodialysis or hemoperfusion for refractory dysrhythmias, hypotension, seizures, or acute very high theophylline levels (>100 μg/mL in acute intoxication, >60 μg/mL in chronic intoxication)

- **Pearl**

Seizures due to theophylline toxicity may be refractory to drug therapy and are associated with worse prognosis; neuromuscular blockade may be necessary in addition to general anesthesia, ventilatory support, and EEG monitoring to control seizures.

Reference

Shannon M: Life-threatening events after theophylline overdose: a 10-year prospective analysis. Arch Intern Med 1999;159:989. [PMID: 10326941]

Tricyclic Antidepressant (TCA) Overdose

- **Essentials of Diagnosis**
  - Constellation of findings reflecting direct CNS, anticholinergic, alpha-adrenergic blockade, direct cardiac effects
  - Mental status varies widely from alert to comatose
  - Anticholinergic: tachycardia, mydriasis, dry skin, urinary retention, ileus, fever, altered mental status, seizures
  - Cardiovascular: tachycardia, dysrhythmias, atrioventricular block
  - Hypotension due to decreased cardiac contractility and alpha-adrenergic blockade
  - ECG valuable for evaluating suspected TCA overdose; common findings include tachycardia, PR and QT prolongation, nonspecific ST changes
  - QRS duration >100 ms suggests serious overdose with potential for significant arrhythmias or seizures; abnormal superior, rightward axis of terminal 40 ms of QRS (wide S in I, aVF and V_6, with prominent R in aVR) strongly suggests TCA overdose and can help discriminate TCA overdose from other drug overdoses

- **Differential Diagnosis**
  - Phenothiazines, anticholinergic, theophylline, beta-blocker, calcium blocker, lidocaine overdose
  - CNS infection
  - Sepsis
  - Hypoglycemia
  - Head trauma

- **Treatment**
  - Cardiac monitor, urinary catheter, IV access
  - Gastric lavage if ingestion within 2 hours, followed by activated charcoal
  - Alkalinization of blood reverses most adverse effects, including hypotension, cardiac arrhythmias, conduction abnormalities
  - Benzodiazepine for agitation or seizures; lidocaine for cardiac arrhythmias unresponsive to bicarbonate

- **Pearl**

Because hypotension is facilitated by alpha-adrenergic blockade, phenylephrine (a pure alpha-adrenergic agonist) is more effective than dopamine for refractory hypotension.

Reference

Kerr GW et al: Tricyclic antidepressant overdose: a review. Emerg Med J 2001;18:236. [PMID: 11435353]

Warfarin Poisoning

- **Essentials of Diagnosis**
  - Bleeding from single or multiple sites, with bruising, epistaxis, gingival bleeding, hematuria, hematochezia, hematemesis, menorrhagia
  - Prolonged PT, normal or prolonged PTT, normal thrombin time, normal fibrinogen level
  - Can occur either by ingestion of warfarin (drug) or ingestion of rodenticides containing similar agents (most rodenticides contain small amounts of anticoagulant and rarely associated with significant toxicity)
  - Allopurinol, cephalosporin, cimetidine, tricyclic antidepressant, erythromycin, NSAIDs, ethanol increase anticoagulant actions of warfarin and contribute to toxicity

- **Differential Diagnosis**
  - Other causes of coagulopathy, including liver disease, vitamin K deficiency, disseminated intravascular coagulation, sepsis-related coagulopathy

- **Treatment**
  - Gastric decontamination within 1 hour of ingestion
  - For life-threatening bleeding, immediate reversal with fresh frozen plasma, IV vitamin K
  - For non-life-threatening bleeding, oral or IV vitamin K in patients not requiring long-term anticoagulation
  - For non-life threatening bleeding in patients requiring subsequent long-term anticoagulation, partial correction with fresh frozen plasma
  - For prolonged PT without bleeding, observation alone usually sufficient

- **Pearl**

Warfarin can be associated with several skin abnormalities including urticaria, purple toe syndrome, and skin necrosis.

Reference

Ansell J, et al: Managing oral anticoagulant therapy. Chest 2001;119(1 Suppl):22S. [PMID: 11157641]

17

Environmental Injuries

Carbon Monoxide (CO) Poisoning

■ Essentials of Diagnosis

- Headache, confusion, neuropsychological impairment, generalized malaise, fatigue, nausea, vomiting, chest pain
- Tachycardia, hypotension, focal and non-focal neurological findings; patients do not have cyanosis; if severe, shock, stupor, coma
- Electrocardiogram (ECG) changes of ischemia in susceptible patients
- May be accidental (operation of motor vehicles in enclosed space, malfunctioning furnaces), concomitant with smoke inhalation, deliberate suicide attempt
- Alcohol, drugs associated with poisoning and death; most common poison-related death in United States
- CO binds to tightly to hemoglobin, also increases O_2 affinity to hemoglobin, resulting in impaired O_2 delivery; also may be intracellular toxin

■ Differential Diagnosis

- Drug overdose
- Hypoxemia
- Cyanide toxicity
- Effects of smoke inhalation

■ Treatment

- Supportive care, especially if cardiovascular compromise, smoke inhalation, burns
- High concentration of inhaled oxygen speeds elimination of carbon monoxide (use non-rebreather O_2 mask or endotracheal intubation with 100% O_2)
- Hyperbaric 100% O_2 increases rate of CO elimination; clinical value unclear
- Transfusion of packed red blood cells may be helpful; consider exchange transfusions in severe toxicity

■ Pearl

The pulse oximeter is unable to distinguish carboxyhemoglobin from oxyhemoglobin; blood must be sent for carboxyhemoglobin concentration.

Reference

Gorman D et al: The clinical toxicology of carbon monoxide. Toxicology 2003;187:25. [PMID: 12679050]

Electrical Shock & Lightning Injury

- **Essentials of Diagnosis**
  - Burns: partial or full thickness skin damage
  - Household current shock: transiently unconscious, headache, cramps, fatigue, paralysis, rhabdomyolysis, atrial or ventricular fibrillation, nonspecific ST-T ECG changes
  - Lightning strike: para- or quadriplegia, autonomic instability, hypertension, nonspecific ST-T ECG changes; blunt trauma due to falls; burns typically superficial
  - Degree of injury depends on conducted current of electricity
  - Alternating current (household) more dangerous than direct current (lightning); high voltage injury defined as >1000 volts

- **Differential Diagnosis**
  - Cardiac arrhythmia
  - Thermal or chemical burns
  - Blunt traumatic injury
  - Toxin or smoke inhalation

- **Treatment**
  - Intubation and mechanical ventilation for respiratory compromise
  - Fluid resuscitation
  - Most immediate risk from cardiac arrhythmia, particularly if electric shock passed through the thorax; most arrhythmias self limited, but may require antiarrhythmic drugs
  - Local care for skin wounds; transfer to burn unit if extensive burns
  - Monitor creatine kinase levels for rhabdomyolysis; if present, consider alkalinization of urine

- **Pearl**

Lightning generates massive peak direct current of 20,000–40,000 amperes for 1–3 microseconds. Despite this, patients surviving the immediate event typically have few complications and often only require observation.

Reference

Koumbourlis AC: Electrical injuries. Crit Care Med 2002;30(11 Suppl):S424. [PMID: 12528784]

Frostbite

- **Essentials of Diagnosis**
  - Superficial frostbitten skin and subcutaneous area typically pain-less, numb, blanched; deep frostbite area may have woody ap-pearance
  - Occurs when tissues become frozen; may see line of demarca-tion between frozen and unfrozen areas
  - Severity of frostbite best determined after rewarming; first de-gree with hyperemia, edema, no blisters; second degree adds blisters, pain during rewarming; third degree with skin necro-sis, eschars, hemorrhagic blisters; fourth degree with complete soft tissue, muscle, bone necrosis

- **Differential Diagnosis**
  - Peripheral arterial disease
  - Raynaud disease
  - Necrotizing fasciitis, cellulitis
  - Immersion foot (prolonged exposure to cold water, non-freez-ing injury)

- **Treatment**
  - Limit cold exposure as soon as possible; avoid rewarming if re-freezing likely
  - Rewarm extremities in warm water bath between 40–42°C; con-tinue rewarming until all blanched tissues perfused with blood
  - Opioid analgesics for pain during rewarming; epidural block during lower extremity rewarming can be used
  - Débride white-blistered tissue after rewarming
  - Aloe vera, applied topically every 6 hours to affected areas, and ibuprofen both inhibit thromboxane; may reduce tissue injury
  - Antibiotic prophylaxis, usually with penicillin, for 48–72 hours
  - Avoid amputation until amount of tissue loss clearly defined; may be weeks or months after injury
  - Treat likely concomitant hypothermia

- **Pearl**

Frostbite rarely occurs unless environmental temperature is less than −6.7°C (20°F).

Reference

Murphy JV et al: Frostbite: pathogenesis and treatment. J Trauma 2000;48:171.
[PMID: 10647591]

Heat Stroke

- **Essentials of Diagnosis**
  - Confusion, stupor, seizures, coma
  - Hot dry skin, hypovolemia, hypotension, tachycardia, body temperature approaching 40°C or more
  - Rhabdomyolysis, myocardial depression, disseminated intravascular coagulation, platelet dysfunction with bleeding, renal failure; intracerebral hemorrhages and cerebral edema may occur
  - Elevated hematocrit, potassium, creatine kinase, prolonged coagulation times
  - Failure of thermoregulatory mechanism.
  - Hyperthermia and CNS dysfunction must be present

- **Differential Diagnosis**
  - Sepsis
  - Neuroleptic malignant syndrome
  - Malignant hyperthermia

- **Treatment**
  - Intubation, mechanical ventilation if patient unconscious.
  - IV fluids
  - Rapid reduction of body temperature to 39°C, using surface cooling with ice, ice water, cooling blankets, water plus fans
  - May also use cold IV fluids, cold water gastric or rectal lavage, peritoneal dialysis with cold fluid
  - Once temperature down to 38°C, cease active cooling measures to avoid hypothermia
  - Multiple organ dysfunction may occur after normalization of temperature and should be managed using standard therapies

- **Pearl**

Acetaminophen and other antipyretics are ineffective in heat stroke, as the hyperthermia in heat stroke is not due to an increase in temperature regulatory set point, as it is in other causes of fever.

Reference

Bouchama A et al: Heat stroke. N Engl J Med 2002;346:1978. [PMID: 12075060]

Hypothermia

■ Essentials of Diagnosis

- Mild (32.2–35°C): shivering, confusion, slurred speech, amnesia, tachycardia, tachypnea
- Moderate (28–32.2°C): decreased shivering, muscle rigidity, lethargy, hallucinations, dilated pupils, bradycardia, hypotension, ventricular arrhythmias, J wave on ECG, hypoventilation
- Severe (<28°C): coma, hypotension, apnea, ventricular fibrillation, asystole, pulmonary edema, pseudo-rigor mortis (appearance of death)
- Measure core temperature with rectal thermometer capable of recording as low as 25°C
- Usually from exposure; with advanced age, alcoholism

■ Differential Diagnosis

- Drug and alcohol intoxication
- Hypothyroidism, adrenal insufficiency
- Sepsis, trauma, burns

■ Treatment

- Remove wet clothing, protect against further heat loss
- Continuous cardiac monitoring; avoid excessive movement of patient, which can trigger arrhythmias
- Intubation and mechanical ventilation
- IV fluids, as most volume depleted; in moderate to severe hypothermia, warm intravenous fluids to 40–42°C
- Defibrillate for pulseless ventricular rhythm; if unsuccessful, rewarm, defibrillate after every 1–2°C increase
- Bradycardia, atrial fibrillation often respond to rewarming
- Antiarrhythmics, vasopressors usually ineffective below 30°C
- Mild hypothermia: passive external rewarming with blankets
- Moderate to severe hypothermia: passive external plus active external rewarming (immersion in 40°C bath, radiant heat, heating pads, warmed forced air)
- Severe hypothermia: active core rewarming with heated humidified oxygen, peritoneal irrigation or pleural or gastric lavage; consider extracorporeal blood rewarming

■ Pearl

The hypothermic patient has potential for full recovery once rewarmed despite severely depressed cardiac function.

Reference

Hanania NA et al: Accidental hypothermia. Crit Care Clin 1999;15:235. [PMID: 10331126]

Mushroom Poisoning

■ Essentials of Diagnosis

- Cyclopeptides (including *Amanita phalloides*, *Galerina marginata*): 6–12 hours after ingestion, colicky abdominal pain, profuse diarrhea, nausea, vomiting; latent phase for 3–5 days, then hepatic toxicity phase with liver failure
- Gyromitrins: 6–12 hours post ingestion, gastritis, dizziness, bloating, nausea, vomiting, headache; if severe, hepatic failure 3–4 days after ingestion; seizure, coma
- Other mushrooms cause symptoms early, usually 1–2 hours; several cause hallucinations, altered perceptions, drowsiness
- 50% of ingestions and 95% of deaths from cyclopeptide group; gyromitrin responsible for remainder of fatal ingestions

■ Differential Diagnosis

- Gastroenteritis
- Infectious diarrhea
- Hepatic failure (acetaminophen toxicity, viral hepatitis, alcohol)

■ Treatment

- Gastric emptying if <4 hours after ingestion; repeated-dose activated charcoal if after 4 hours.
- Supportive care for hepatic failure; if severe, liver transplantation
- Thioctic acid, silybin, penicillin G, N-acetylcysteine used in cyclopeptide group toxicity; benefit not validated
- Methylene blue for methemoglobinemia associated with gyromitrin group; pyridoxine for refractory seizures

■ Pearl

Of the 500 species of mushrooms in the United States, 100 are toxic and 10 are potentially fatal.

Reference

Enjalbert F et al: Treatment of amatoxin poisoning: 20-year retrospective analysis. J Toxicol Clin Toxicol 2002;40:715. [PMID: 12475187]

Near Drowning

- **Essentials of Diagnosis**
  - Fresh water near-drowning associated with hypervolemia, hypotonicity, dilution of serum electrolytes, intravascular hemolysis
  - Saltwater near-drowning may have hypovolemia, hypertonicity, hemoconcentration
  - Both with hypoxemia, metabolic acidosis, hypothermia; acute respiratory distress syndrome in 50%; cardiac arrhythmias due to hypoxia, acidosis, electrolyte abnormalities
  - Renal failure, disseminated intravascular coagulation, rhabdomyolysis may occur

- **Differential Diagnosis**
  - In SCUBA divers, consider arterial air embolism syndrome, pulmonary barotrauma (pneumothorax)

- **Treatment**
  - Early intubation and mechanical ventilation
  - Aggressive volume resuscitation for hypotension
  - Correct electrolyte abnormalities
  - Supportive care for complications such as renal failure, rhabdomyolysis, disseminated intravascular coagulation, hypothermia, aspiration pneumonia

- **Pearl**

Intoxication with alcohol or drugs is a factor in more than half of near drowning cases.

Reference

Bierens JJ et al: Drowning. Curr Opin Crit Care 2002;8:578. [PMID: 12454545]

Radiation Injury

- **Essentials of Diagnosis**
  - Exposure to accidental or deliberately released material producing ionizing radiation
  - Severity related to dose and duration of exposure; more severe if same dose received over shorter period
  - Acute radiation syndrome (ARS) responsible for most deaths in first 60 days after exposure; damage to gastrointestinal, hematologic, cardiovascular, central nervous systems
  - ARS severity dose-dependent: <2 grays (Gy)—minimal symptoms, mild reduction in platelets and granulocytes after 30 day latent period; 2–4 Gy—transient nausea, vomiting 1–4 hours after exposure; after 1–3 weeks, nausea, vomiting, bloody diarrhea, bone marrow depression; 6–10 Gy—severe GI symptoms, severe hematologic complications; >10 Gy, fulminating course with vomiting, diarrhea, dehydration, circulatory collapse, ataxia, confusion, seizures, coma, death

- **Differential Diagnosis**
  - Sepsis
  - Gastroenteritis
  - Hematologic malignancy, aplastic anemia

- **Treatment**
  - Decontamination at or near the site of exposure; removing clothing, washing with soap and water achieves 95% decontamination; decontaminate wounds; remove inhaled or ingested radiation sources
  - Patient should be isolated
  - Prodromal symptoms usually require no treatment; latent period of 1–3 weeks
  - Transfuse blood products as needed
  - If immunosuppression develops, prophylactic antibiotics directed against gastrointestinal organisms may be useful
  - For ARS with exposure >2 Gy, consider possible use of stem cell transfusion, colony stimulating factors

- **Pearl**

Lymphocytes are the most sensitive cells to radiation injury. The pattern of lymphocyte decline over the first 24 hours after exposure can provide an estimate of radiation dose received by referring to standard lymphocyte depletion curves.

Reference

Mettler FA Jr, Voelz GL: Major radiation exposure—what to expect and how to respond. N Engl J Med 2002;346:1554. [PMID: 12015396]

Snakebite

- **Essentials of Diagnosis**
  - 95% of poisonous bites from Crotalidae or pit vipers, including rattlesnakes, cottonmouths, copperheads; 5% from Elapidae (coral snakes)
  - Crotalid envenomations: swelling, erythema, ecchymosis, perioral paresthesias, coagulopathy, hypotension, tachypnea, and respiratory compromise; bites characterized by two fang marks
  - Elapidae envenomations: delayed 1–12 hours, include paralysis, respiratory compromise
  - Severity of envenomation estimated by rate of progression of signs, symptoms, coagulopathy; mild with only local effects; moderate with non-severe systemic effects, minimal coagulopathy; severe with life-threatening hypotension, altered sensorium, severe coagulopathy and thrombocytopenia

- **Differential Diagnosis**
  - Sepsis
  - Insect or spider bites
  - Toxin or chemical ingestion or inhalation

- **Treatment**
  - Maintain airway in bites of head and neck, or when respiratory compromise present
  - Fluid resuscitation for hypotension
  - Two crotalid antivenoms available: Antivenom (Crotalidae) Polyvalent (ACP) and newer Crotalidae Polyvalent Immune Fab Ovine (FabAV); antivenom recommended for crotalid envenomations with severe signs and symptoms or with progression, particularly coagulopathy or hemolysis
  - Give ACP slowly: 2–4 vials for minimal envenomation, 5–9 vials for moderate, 10–15 for severe; perform skin test with ACP before administration to predict allergic reaction; 15–20% with moderate to severe antivenom reactions (treat with diphenhydramine and antihistamines)
  - Reactions infrequent with FabAV; administer 3–12 vials initially, followed by 2 vials at 6, 12, and 18 hours
  - Watch extremities for evidence of compartment syndrome

- **Pearl**

To distinguish between bites of the poisonous coral snake and non-poisonous king snake, use this mnemonic: "red on yellow (coral), kills a fellow; red on black (king), venom lack."

Reference

Gold BS et al: Bites of venomous snakes. N Engl J Med 2002;347:347. [PMID: 12151473]

Spider & Scorpion Bites

- **Essentials of Diagnosis**
  - Black widow spider bite initially painless, after 10–60 minutes, pain, muscle spasms, headache, nausea, vomiting, rigidity of abdominal wall; symptoms peak 2–3 hours after bite, may persist 24 hours
  - Brown recluse spider bites have pain 1–4 hours after bite, erythema with pustule or bull's-eye pattern; ulcer may form after several days; rarely systemic reactions 1–2 days later, including hemolysis, hemoglobinuria, jaundice, renal failure, pulmonary edema, disseminated intravascular coagulation
  - Scorpion bites cause severe pain without erythema, swelling; rare systemic reactions include restlessness, jerking, nystagmus, hypertension, diplopia, confusion, seizures

- **Differential Diagnosis**
  - Acute abdomen (black widow spider)
  - Insect bites, including ticks
  - Staphylococcal, streptococcal skin infections
  - Chronic herpes simplex, varicella-zoster
  - Vasculitis, other skin disorders

- **Treatment**
  - Black widow spider bites: pain relief with intravenous opioids, antivenom in severe cases, supportive care if organ failure
  - Brown recluse spider bites: ice to local area, supportive care, debridement if severe ulceration forms at bite area
  - Scorpion bites: ice to local area; antivenom in severe cases; do not use opioids, as they might potentiate venom toxicity

- **Pearl**

When trying to determine if bite is from a spider or other type of insect, spiders usually only bite once, whereas other insects bite multiple times.

Reference

Anderson PC: Spider bites in the United States. Dermatol Clin 1997;15:307. [PMID: 9098639]

18

Dermatology

Candidiasis (Moniliasis)

- **Essentials of Diagnosis**
  - Mucosal candidiasis: white, curd-like plaques on oral or vaginal mucosa, uncircumcised penis (balanitis); red, macerated base, with painful erosions; oral infection may spread to angles of mouth (angular cheilitis), with fissuring of oral commissures
  - Cutaneous candidiasis: easily ruptured pustules in intertriginous areas (groin, under breasts, abdominal folds); with rupture of pustules, bright red base seen, with moist scale at borders; intense pruritus, irritation and burning
  - Diagnosis established with potassium hydroxide preparation demonstrating budding yeast or spores and pseudohyphae

- **Differential Diagnosis**
  - Oral candidiasis: leukoplakia, coated tongue
  - Cutaneous candidiasis: eczematous eruptions, dermatophytosis, bacterial skin infections (pyodermas)

- **Treatment**
  - Keep moist areas clean and dry
  - Apply topical anticandidal creams (e.g., clotrimazole) twice a day
  - Low-potency topical steroid may reduce inflammatory component

- **Pearl**

Patients with mucosal candidiasis should be evaluated for predisposing condition such as diabetes, malignancy, HIV.

Reference

Vazquez JA, Sobel JD: Mucosal candidiasis. Infect Dis Clin North Am 2002;16:793. [PMID: 12512182]

Contact Dermatitis

- **Essentials of Diagnosis**
  - Circumscribed vesiculobullous eruptions on erythematous base, confined to area of contact
  - History of exposure or contact to allergen or irritant
  - Linear pattern or characteristic configuration suggesting external contact
  - Pruritus may be prominent symptom

- **Differential Diagnosis**
  - Other eczematous eruptions
  - Impetigo
  - Cutaneous candidiasis

- **Treatment**
  - Remove suspected irritant or allergen
  - Apply high-potency topical steroid cream twice daily to affected area
  - Use low- or medium-potency topical steroid for face or intertriginous areas
  - Antihistamines to control itching

- **Pearl**

Any substance in contact with skin (tape, soap, body fluid, topical medication, even steroid cream) may be offending agent.

Reference

Rietchel RL, Fowler JF Jr: Fisher's Contact Dermatitis, 5th ed. Lippincott Williams & Wilkins, 2001.

Disseminated Intravascular Coagulation (DIC) & Purpura Fulminans

- **Essentials of Diagnosis**
  - Ranges from mild bruising and oozing at venipuncture sites to massive hemorrhage and necrosis accompanying abnormal bleeding or clotting as result of uncontrolled activation of co-agulation and fibrinolysis
  - Purpura fulminans characterized by acute, rapidly enlarging, tender, irregular areas of purpura, especially over extremities; may evolve into hemorrhagic bullae with necrosis and eschar formation
  - Excessive generation of thrombin, formation of intravascular fibrin clots, consumption of platelets and coagulation factors
  - Laboratory findings: thrombocytopenia, anemia, prolonged pro-thrombin and partial thromboplastin times, low fibrinogen, increased fibrin degradation products
  - May be accompanied by pulmonary, hepatic, or renal failure, gastrointestinal bleeding, and hemorrhagic adrenal infarction

- **Differential Diagnosis**
  - Severe liver disease
  - Thrombotic thrombocytopenic purpura
  - Vitamin K deficiency
  - Heparin-induced thrombocytopenia
  - Congenital or acquired protein S or C deficiency
  - Microangiopathic hemolytic anemias
  - Acute promyelocytic leukemia (M3 variant)

- **Treatment**
  - Hemodynamic stabilization
  - Treatment of underlying infection/disorder
  - Transfusion of fresh frozen plasma, cryoprecipitate
  - Heparin rarely indicated

- **Pearl**

Clinically overt disseminated intravascular coagulopathy (DIC) is as common in patients with gram-positive sepsis as in those with gram-negative sepsis.

Reference

Levi M et al: Disseminated intravascular coagulation. N Engl J Med 1999;341:586. [PMID: 1045465]

Erythema Multiforme & Stevens-Johnson Syndrome

- **Essentials of Diagnosis**
  - Erythema multiforme: hypersensitivity reaction to medications and infectious agents
  - Low-grade fever, malaise, upper respiratory symptoms, followed by nonspecific symmetric eruption of erythematous macules, papules, urticarial plaques
  - Evolves into concentric rings of erythema with papular, dusky, necrotic or bullous centers ("target lesions") over 1–2 days
  - May also appear as annular, polycyclic, or purpuric lesions (multiforme)
  - Stevens-Johnson syndrome: high fever, headache, myalgias, sore throat (>1 mucosal surface affected), with conspicuous stomatitis, beginning with vesicles on lips, tongue, buccal mucosa, rapidly evolving into erosions and ulcers covered by hemorrhagic crusts

- **Differential Diagnosis**
  - Erythema multiforme without classic target lesions: urticarial eruptions, viral exanthems, vasculitis
  - Mucocutaneous ulcerations: Reiter syndrome, Behçet syndrome, herpes gingivostomatitis
  - Bullous impetigo, bullous pemphigoid, pemphigus vulgaris, toxic epidermal necrolysis

- **Treatment**
  - Supportive care, symptomatic therapy, optimize nutrition
  - Discontinue potential offending agents
  - Monitor closely for progression to secondary bacterial infection or toxic epidermal necrolysis

- **Pearl**

Erythema multiforme occurs in all age groups, while Stevens-Johnson syndrome most often affects children and young men.

Reference

Prendiville J: Stevens-Johnson syndrome and toxic epidermal necrolysis. Adv Dermatol 2002;18:151. [PMID: 12528405]

Exfoliative Erythroderma

- **Essentials of Diagnosis**
  - Generalized diffuse erythema with scaling, induration, variable desquamation; mucous membranes usually spared
  - Pruritus, malaise, fever, chills and weight loss may be present; thermoregulatory dysfunction may lead to relative hypothermia and chills; excoriations, peripheral edema, lymphadenopathy common
  - Leukocytosis and anemia; eosinophilia suggestive of underlying drug reaction
  - Caused by multiple underlying conditions including eczematous conditions, psoriasis, scabies, medications, lymphoma
  - Skin biopsy results often nonspecific; may reveal cutaneous T cell lymphoma, leukemia, Norwegian crusted scabies

- **Differential Diagnosis**
  - Morbilliform drug eruptions
  - Viral exanthems
  - Early phase of toxic epidermal necrolysis
  - Toxic shock syndrome
  - Graft-versus-host disease

- **Treatment**
  - Symptomatic relief; specific therapy once etiology known
  - Optimize nutrition
  - Discontinue possible offending agents
  - Avoid systemic steroids unless indicated as specific therapy for underlying disease
  - Daily whirlpool treatments to remove scale; apply medium potency topical steroid cream

- **Pearl**

Serologic testing for HIV is recommended in all patients with erythrodermic psoriasis.

Reference

Rothe MJ et al: Erythroderma. Dermatol Clin 2000;18:405. [PMID: 10943536]

Generalized Pustular Psoriasis

- **Essentials of Diagnosis**
  - Serious, potentially fatal form of psoriasis occurring in patients over age 40
  - Acute onset of widespread erythematous areas studded with pustules, with accompanying fever, chills, leukocytosis
  - Recurrent waves of pustulation and remission occur
  - Mouth and tongue commonly involved
  - Precipitating events: topical and systemic corticosteroid therapy or withdrawal, medications (sulfonamides, penicillin, lithium, pyrazolones), infections, pregnancy, hypocalcemia
  - Complications: bacterial superinfection, arthritis, pericholangitis, circulatory shunting with accompanying hypotension, high-output heart failure, and renal failure

- **Differential Diagnosis**
  - Miliaria rubra
  - Secondary syphilis
  - Pustular drug eruption
  - Folliculitis

- **Treatment**
  - Retinoids, acitretin, and isotretinoin drugs of choice, but should be avoided in persons with hepatitis, lipid abnormalities; most show improvement in 5–7 days
  - Methotrexate, cyclosporine alternatives in select cases
  - Avoid systemic steroids

- **Pearl**

HIV testing should be carried out in all patients with psoriasis, as severe psoriatic exacerbations occur in HIV-infected individuals.

Reference

Mengesha YM, Bennett ML: Pustular skin disorders: diagnosis and treatment. Am J Clin Dermatol 2002;3:389. [PMID: 12113648]

Graft-Versus-Host Disease (GVHD)

- ■ Essentials of Diagnosis
  - • Prior allogeneic transplant of immunologically competent cells, particularly bone marrow, reacts against host tissue
  - • Acute GVHD (days to weeks following transplant): Pruritic macular and papular erythema, beginning on palms, soles, ears, upper trunk, frequently progressing to generalized erythroderma with bullae in severe cases; incidence 10–80%; extracutaneous manifestations of GVHD (diarrhea, hepatitis, delayed immunologic recovery) follow skin eruption
  - • Total bilirubin, stool output, and severity of rash are prognostic factors
  - • Chronic GVHD (50–100 days following transplant): Widespread scaly plaques and desquamation; cicatricial alopecia, dystrophic nails, and sometimes sclerodermatous changes supervene; incidence 30–60%

- ■ Differential Diagnosis
  - • Acute GVHD: toxic epidermal necrolysis, drug-induced eruptions, infectious exanthems
  - • Chronic GVHD: scleroderma, lupus erythematosus, dermatomyositis

- ■ Treatment
  - • Prevention of GVHD with immunomodulating agents
  - • Irradiate blood products prior to transfusion
  - • Acute and chronic GVH may respond to increased immunosuppression
  - • Photochemotherapy with oral psoralen (PUVA) or UVA sometimes used

- ■ Pearl

The skin is the most commonly affected organ in acute graft-versus-host disease.

Reference

Vargas-Diez E et al: Analysis of risk factors for acute cutaneous graft-versus-host disease after allogeneic stem cell transplantation. Br J Dermatol 2003;148:1129. [PMID: 12828739]

Meningococcemia

- **Essentials of Diagnosis**
  - *Neisseria meningitidis*: gram-negative diplococcus causing spectrum of diseases, most commonly in children under age 15
  - Incubation period 2–10 days; insidious or abrupt onset
  - Petechial rash on trunk, lower extremities, palms, soles and mucous membranes; rash may be urticarial or morbilliform
  - May be complicated by purpura fulminans, with extensive hemorrhagic bullae and areas of necrosis
  - Other complications include meningitis, arthritis, myocarditis, pericarditis, acute adrenal infarction, hypotension, shock
  - Diagnosis confirmed by demonstrating organism by Gram stain or culture (blood, cerebrospinal fluid (CSF), skin lesion) or by serologic testing

- **Differential Diagnosis**
  - Sepsis or meningitis caused by other bacteria
  - Rocky Mountain spotted fever
  - Viral infections (echovirus, coxsackievirus, atypical measles)
  - Vasculitis

- **Treatment**
  - Supportive care with attention to maintaining blood pressure and organ perfusion
  - Intravenous penicillin or ceftriaxone

- **Pearl**

Respiratory isolation is mandatory for suspected meningococcal disease; consider ciprofloxacin or rifampin for close contacts of patients with intimate exposure.

Reference

Stephens DS, Zimmer SM: Pathogenesis, therapy, and prevention of meningococcal sepsis. Curr Infect Dis Rep 2002;4:377. [PMID: 12228024]

Miliaria (Heat Rash)

- **Essentials of Diagnosis**
  - Common disorder characterized by retention of sweat in bedridden patients with fever and increased sweating
  - Miliaria crystallina: small, superficial sweat-filled vesicles that rupture easily, without surrounding inflammation ("dew-drops" on skin)
  - Miliaria rubra (prickly heat): discrete, pruritic, erythematous papules and vesiculopustules on back, chest, antecubital and popliteal fossae
  - Burning, itching, superficial small vesicles, papules or pustules on covered areas of the skin

- **Differential Diagnosis**
  - Folliculitis (miliaria rubra)

- **Treatment**
  - Keep patient cool and dry
  - Symptomatic treatment for pruritus

- **Pearl**

Obstruction of eccrine sweat glands leads to formation of miliaria.

Reference

Feng E et al: Miliaria. Cutis 1995;55:213. [PMID: 7796612]

Morbilliform, Urticarial, & Bullous Drug Reactions

- ### Essentials of Diagnosis
  - Onset of rash 5–10 days after exposure to new drug, or 1–2 days following re-exposure to drug to which a patient has been sensitized; occurs in 25–30% of hospitalized patients
  - Usually symmetric, widespread, with pruritus and low grade fever; resolution of rash when drug discontinued supports diagnosis
  - Morbilliform eruptions most common form of drug-induced rash; usually begins on trunk or dependent areas
  - Urticaria characterized by pink, edematous, pruritic wheals of varying size and shape, usually lasting less than 24 hours
  - Angioedema represents urticarial involvement of deep dermal and subcutaneous tissues, sometimes involving mucous membranes
  - Bullous drug eruptions include fixed-drug eruptions, erythema multiforme, Stevens-Johnson syndrome, toxic epidermal necrolysis, vasculitis, and anticoagulant necrosis

- ### Differential Diagnosis
  - Morbilliform eruption: bacterial or rickettsial infection, or collagen-vascular disease
  - Non–drug-associated urticarial eruptions: food allergies, insect bites or stings, parasitic infections, and vasculitis or serum-sickness
  - Bullous drug eruptions: primary bullous dermatoses (bullous pemphigoid, porphyria cutanea tarda)

- ### Treatment
  - Identify and discontinue likely causative agents; substitute chemically unrelated alternatives
  - Morbilliform eruptions: supportive measures, symptomatic treatment (oral antihistamine, topical anti-pruritic agent)
  - Urticarial eruptions: if severe, aggressive supportive measures to support blood pressure; epinephrine, fluids, antihistamines, sometimes corticosteroids
  - Blistering eruptions: decompress large bullae; topical compresses to remove exudates or crusts

- ### Pearl
  Drug eruptions are most commonly associated with antibiotics, anticonvulsants, and blood products.

Reference
Nigen S et al: Drug eruptions: approaching the diagnosis of drug-induced skin diseases. J Drugs Dermatol 2003;2:278. [PMID: 12848112]

Pemphigus Vulgaris

- **Essentials of Diagnosis**
  - Flaccid, easily ruptured blisters on noninflamed skin; after rupture, nonhealing crusted erosions remain; > 50% begin with painful oral erosions
  - Superficial detachment of skin after pressure or trauma (Nikolsky sign)
  - Skin biopsy: characteristic intraepidermal cleft just above basal cell layer with separation of keratinocytes from one another (acantholysis)
  - Direct immunofluorescence of normal-appearing skin shows intercellular IgG and complement throughout epithelium
  - Rare, life-threatening disease (mortality rate 60—90% before; 10% after advent of corticosteroids) caused by circulating IgG autoantibodies directed against intercellular substance of epidermis

- **Differential Diagnosis**
  - Erythema multiforme, Stevens-Johnson syndrome, toxic epidermal necrolysis
  - Bullous drug eruptions
  - Bullous impetigo
  - Other primary blistering diseases (bullous pemphigoid, dermatitis herpetiformis)

- **Treatment**
  - Discontinue drugs known to be associated with pemphigus (penicillamine, captopril)
  - Prednisone, 60–120 mg/d, in combination with azathioprine, 100–150 mg/d, usually effective
  - Prior to therapy, patient should be evaluated for contraindications to systemic steroids
  - When control of the blistering is achieved, prednisone is gradually reduced as tolerated
  - Methotrexate, cyclophosphamide, mycophenolate mofetil, cyclosporine, gold, plasmapheresis alternative modalities
  - Whirlpool treatments helpful in removing crusts from lesions
  - Oral mucosal erosions may benefit from topical steroids, antiseptics, viscous lidocaine, attention to oral hygiene

- **Pearl**

Paraneoplastic pemphigus is a very rare complication of cancer, most often non-Hodgkin's lymphoma, with overlapping clinical and histological features to pemphigus vulgaris.

Reference

Fellner MJ, Sapadin AN: Current therapy of pemphigus vulgaris. Mt Sinai J Med 2001;68(4-5):268. [PMID: 11514914]

Phenytoin Hypersensitivity Syndrome

- ■ Essentials of Diagnosis
  - • High spiking fever, malaise, rash 2–3 weeks after starting phenytoin therapy; sooner if prior exposure to drug
  - • Patchy erythematous rash evolving into extensive pruritic maculopapular rash, occasionally with follicular papules and pustules; may evolve to exfoliative erythroderma, erythema multiforme, Stevens-Johnson syndrome, toxic epidermal necrolysis
  - • Edema of palms, soles, and face
  - • Tender localized or generalized lymphadenopathy
  - • Mild to severe hepatic injury; mortality up to 20% with severe liver damage
  - • Sometimes conjunctivitis, pharyngitis, diarrhea, myositis, and reversible acute renal failure
  - • Leukocytosis with eosinophilia (5–50%); normal erythrocyte sedimentation rate, serum complement
  - • Adverse skin reactions in 3–15% of patients receiving phenytoin; smaller percentage develop syndrome of rash, fever, eosinophilia, hepatic injury
  - • All age groups affected; incidence highest in blacks; likely immune-mediated

- ■ Differential Diagnosis
  - • Infectious mononucleosis
  - • Other anticonvulsant medication reactions with rash and multisystemic involvement (phenobarbital)
  - • Other drug reactions
  - • Vasculitis

- ■ Treatment
  - • Medication must be discontinued
  - • Cross-reactivity among anticonvulsants possible; valproic acid or carbamazepine may be safer alternatives
  - • General supportive care, especially with multisystem involvement
  - • No demonstrated benefit of systemic corticosteroids

- ■ Pearl

In patients with anticonvulsant hypersensitivity syndrome to either phenytoin, phenobarbital or carbamazepine, up to 75% have demonstrated in vitro cross sensitivity to the other two drugs.

Reference

Schlienger RG, Shear NH: Antiepileptic drug hypersensitivity syndrome. Epilepsia 1998;39 (7 Suppl:)S3-7. [PMID: 9798755]

Rocky Mountain Spotted Fever

- Essentials of Diagnosis
  - Acute systemic illness with fever and purpuric eruption
  - Caused by *Rickettsia rickettsii*, transmitted by ticks in mid-Atlantic and Rocky Mountain states
  - Highest incidence in spring and summer; 1–14 day incubation period, followed by sudden onset of fever, headache, myalgia, nausea and vomiting
  - May be complicated by central nervous system, cardiac, pulmonary and renal involvement
  - Disseminated intravascular coagulation may lead to shock and death
  - Diagnosis established by serologic tests, often retrospectively; tests are not reliable before second week of illness

- Differential Diagnosis
  - Viral or bacterial meningitis
  - Meningococcemia
  - Measles
  - Vasculitis
  - Thrombotic thrombocytopenic purpura

- Treatment
  - Initiate treatment as soon as diagnosis is suspected with doxycycline or chloramphenicol

- Pearl

Rapidly progressive rash with bilateral symmetric petechiae of the palms and soles are the hallmarks of Rocky Mountain spotted fever.

Reference

Masters EJ et al: Rocky Mountain spotted fever: a clinician's dilemma. Arch Intern Med 2003;163:769. [PMID: 12695267]

Rubeola (Measles)

- **Essentials of Diagnosis**
  - Acute epidemic disease with marked upper respiratory symptoms and widespread erythematous maculopapular rash
  - Incubation period 7–14 days, followed by high fever, cough, coryza, conjunctivitis with photophobia
  - Discrete erythematous macules and thin papules appear on day 3–5, first on forehead and behind ears, coalescing and spreading to trunk and extremities
  - Koplik spots usually appear on buccal mucosa 1–2 days before exanthema
  - Complications: secondary bacterial infection, otitis media, pneumonia, viral myocarditis, liver function abnormalities, and thrombocytopenia

- **Differential Diagnosis**
  - Cutaneous drug reactions
  - Other viral exanthems

- **Treatment**
  - Supportive care
  - No proven antiviral therapy exists for rubeola
  - Aerosolized ribavirin, intravenous immunoglobulin (IGIV), and interferon may be useful for treatment of measles pneumonitis or encephalitis
  - Respiratory isolation precautions

- **Pearl**

The clinical presentation of rubeola in the immunocompromised patients is atypical, with 30–40% having no rash.

Reference

Duke T, Mgone CS Measles: not just another viral exanthem. Lancet 2003;361:763. [PMID: 12620751]

Toxic Epidermal Necrolysis (TEN)

- **■ Essentials of Diagnosis**
  - Rare, life-threatening syndrome characterized by skin tenderness, discrete erythematous macules, and exfoliation of epidermis and mucous membranes
  - Red, scalded appearance of skin; bullae and epidermal sloughing
  - Majority are drug-induced (anticonvulsants, sulfa-containing antibiotics, NSAIDs, allopurinol)
  - Subepidermal separation of skin (Nikolsky sign); not specific
  - Features of Stevens-Johnson syndrome (stomatitis, blotchy eruption with target lesions)
  - Complications: fluid loss, thermoregulatory impairment; sepsis most common cause of death

- **■ Differential Diagnosis**
  - Staphylococcal scalded skin syndrome
  - Pemphigus vulgaris, other blistering diseases
  - Toxic shock syndrome
  - Chemical or thermal burns
  - Kawasaki disease
  - Stevens-Johnson syndrome

- **■ Treatment**
  - Manage as extensive second degree burns, ideally in burn unit
  - Discontinue most likely offending medication
  - Pain control
  - Aggressive repletion of fluids, electrolytes, nutritional support (enteral feeding preferred over parenteral nutrition)
  - Avoid prophylactic antibiotics to prevent emergence of resistant bacteria
  - Ophthalmologic consultation critical to avoid ocular sequelae

- **■ Pearl**

Avoid silver sulfadiazine in patients with toxic epidermal necrolysis and suspected sulfonamide sensitivity.

Reference

Nigen S et al: Drug eruptions: approaching the diagnosis of drug-induced skin diseases. J Drugs Dermatol 2003;2:278. [PMID: 12848112]

Toxic Shock Syndrome

- **Essentials of Diagnosis**
  - Multisystem illness characterized by rapid onset of fever, vomiting, watery diarrhea, pharyngitis, profound myalgias with accompanying hypotension
  - Diffuse blanching truncal erythema early, accentuated in axillary and inguinal folds, spreading to extremities; desquamation of skin, palms and soles occurs in second or third week
  - Multi-organ system involvement, with acute renal failure, acute respiratory distress syndrome (ARDS), refractory shock, ventricular arrhythmias, and DIC may occur
  - Highest incidence in menstruating women, persons with localized or post-surgical staphylococcal infection, and women using diaphragm or contraceptive sponge

- **Differential Diagnosis**
  - Scarlet fever/Streptococcal toxic shock-like disease
  - Kawasaki disease
  - Rocky Mountain spotted fever
  - Drug eruptions/Stevens-Johnson syndrome
  - Measles
  - Leptospirosis
  - Sepsis syndrome with multi-organ system failure

- **Treatment**
  - Immediate removal of tampon, contraceptive device, or surgical packing
  - Surgical drainage, irrigation of focal abscess
  - Supportive care, with fluid resuscitation and management of organ system failure
  - Anti-staphylococcal antibiotic, though effect on outcome unclear

- **Pearl**

Intense hyperemia of conjunctival, oropharyngeal, and vaginal surfaces are frequent findings in toxic shock syndrome.

Reference

Provost TT, Flynn JA (editors): Cutaneous medicine: Cutaneous manifestations of systemic disease. BC Decker, 2001.

Varicella-Zoster Virus (VZV)

- **Essentials of Diagnosis**
  - Varicella-zoster virus: herpes virus causing two syndromes, primary varicella and herpes zoster infection (shingles)
  - Primary varicella: 11–21 day incubation period with ensuing 1–3 day mild prodrome of fever, malaise; small, erythematous macules appear on trunk, face, with centripetal spread to extremities; formation of clear vesicles which rupture and crust over; oropharyngeal vesicles rupture quickly to form superficial mucosal ulcers
  - Complications of primary varicella: hepatitis, pneumonitis, myocarditis, encephalitis, and DIC
  - Diagnosis by demonstration of multinucleated giant cells on Tzanck smear; confirmed by immunofluorescent antibody stain or culture
  - Reactivation infection: acute, often painful unilateral eruption in dermatomal distribution, with clusters of vesicles on erythematous base

- **Differential Diagnosis**
  - Extensive impetigo
  - Disseminated herpes simplex infection
  - Eczema herpeticum

- **Treatment**
  - Treat all VZV infections in immunocompromised host with IV acyclovir (10 mg/kg q 8h, 7–10 days)
  - Primary varicella in teenagers and adults: oral acyclovir (800 mg PO five times daily for 5–7 days)
  - Varicella zoster in elderly: if lesions present < 72 hours, give 7 days course of oral acyclovir, famciclovir or valacyclovir
  - Treat secondary bacterial infection when present
  - Symptomatic treatment with cool compresses, antihistamines

- **Pearl**

In immunocompromised persons, herpes zoster lesions may disseminate widely, or become necrotic, hemorrhagic, or both.

Reference

Chen TM et al: Clinical manifestations of varicella-zoster virus infection. Dermatol Clin 2002;20(2):267. [PMID: 12120440]

19

Oncology/Oncologic Emergencies

Leukemia, Acute

- ■ Essentials of Diagnosis
  - Pancytopenia: weakness, fatigue from anemia; bleeding (gingival, epistaxis) from thrombocytopenia; infection from ineffective leukocytes
  - No characteristic examination findings; fever; pallor, petechiae, retinal hemorrhages, gingival hypertrophy (monocytic subtypes), lymphadenopathy and splenomegaly (acute lymphoblastic leukemia, evolution from chronic myelogenous leukemia); rarely extramedullary leukemic involvement (chloroma)
  - Peripheral blood smear may have no, little, or marked increase in white blood cells; thrombocytopenia; >30% blasts in bone marrow
  - Distinguish acute myelogenous leukemia (AML) from acute lymphoblastic leukemia (ALL) by Auer rods (AML), histochemical markers; cytogenetics may have prognostic importance
  - AML has 7 subtypes; acute promyelocytic leukemia (APL, AML-M3) associated with disseminated intravascular coagulopathy (DIC), spontaneous hemorrhage

- ■ Differential Diagnosis
  - Aplastic anemia   • Leukemoid reaction
  - Bone marrow infiltration with tumor, microorganisms

- ■ Treatment
  - High-dose chemotherapy based on cell type followed by prolonged pancytopenia requiring aggressive transfusions of red cells, platelets
  - Careful hand washing, avoid intramuscular injections; long-term "tunnel" catheter may be helpful
  - Evaluate neutropenic fever; treat with empiric antibiotics
  - Anticipate tumor lysis syndrome; treat with IV fluids, allopurinol
  - APL may respond to all-trans retinoic acid (ATRA) and chemotherapy
  - Selected patients may benefit from bone marrow transplantation

- ■ Pearl

ATRA treatment of APL may be complicated by retinoic acid syndrome in 6–27%, with fever, weight gain, hypotension, renal failure, pulmonary edema, and pleural and pericardial effusions.

Reference

Massion PB et al: Prognosis of hematologic malignancies does not predict intensive care unit mortality. Crit Care Med 2002;30:2260. [PMID: 12394954]

Spinal Cord Compression

- **Essentials of Diagnosis**
  - Dull aching axial back pain that may radiate to arms or legs; band-like discomfort around chest; worse at night; aggravated by movement
  - Neurologic deficits depend on level of involvement: 70% thoracic, 20% lumbar, 10% cervical; typically begins with motor impairment; high cervical cord lesions may be life-threatening; thoracic cord lesions have truncal sensory level, lower extremity weakness, autonomic dysfunction; lumbosacral cord lesions may have radiculopathy and loss of reflexes or conus syndrome
  - Acquire imaging studies as soon as possible; MRI, or CT myelogram
  - May be first manifestation of malignancy; most common are cancers of lung, breast, prostate, lymphoma, multiple myeloma
  - Epidural spinal cord compression develops from direct metastatic spread of cancer to vertebral body or from paravertebral location with extension into epidural space

- **Differential Diagnosis**
  - Intervertebral disk herniation
  - Benign neoplasms
  - Transverse myelitis
  - Paraneoplastic syndrome
  - Spinal cord infarction
  - Multiple sclerosis
  - Epidural abscess
  - Carcinomatous meningitis

- **Treatment**
  - Corticosteroids should be started as soon as diagnosis suspected; delay may lead to progression of neurologic deficit
  - External beam radiation to involved area
  - Chemotherapy based on underlying malignancy
  - Surgery indicated for spinal instability or bone deformity, failure to respond to radiation therapy, radioresistant tumor, atlantoaxial compression, solitary spinal cord metastasis
  - Monitor changes in neurologic exam closely

- **Pearl**

Epidural spinal cord compression should be considered in any patient with cancer and axial skeletal pain as pain is the most common early symptom.

Reference

Daw HA et al: Epidural spinal cord compression in cancer patients: diagnosis and management. Cleve Clin J Med 2000;67:497. [PMID: 10902239]

Superior Vena Cava (SVC) Syndrome

- **Essentials of Diagnosis**
  - Compression, invasion, or thrombosis of SVC; most commonly caused by malignancy
  - Headache, dizziness, sensation of fullness in head
  - Distention of neck and anterior chest wall veins
  - Facial plethora and edema
  - Cyanosis and edema of upper extremities
  - Dyspnea may occur from airway compression
  - Diagnosis made on clinical grounds in majority of cases
  - Chest radiographs, tomography, CT scans define extent of mediastinal involvement
  - Tissue diagnosis needed to establish etiology and guide therapeutic options
  - Etiologies: malignancy with lung cancer and lymphoma most common; benign causes include aortic aneurysm, fibrosing mediastinitis, tuberculosis, pyogenic infection, radiation changes; thrombotic complications from intravascular catheters

- **Differential Diagnosis**
  - Angioedema
  - Histoplasmosis
  - Upper extremity deep vein thrombosis
  - Thyroid goiter
  - Syphilitic aneurysm of aorta

- **Treatment**
  - Chemotherapy treatment of choice for small cell lung cancer, lymphoma, germ cell tumors
  - Radiation therapy only option for all other tumors
  - Symptom relief measures: elevating head of bed, oxygen
  - Secure patency of airway with stents if needed to prevent tracheal compression
  - Corticosteroids may help decrease edema and secondary inflammatory reaction
  - Saphenous vein bypass grafting useful in selected patients
  - Diuretics, anticoagulants, thrombolytic agents are of little help and may actually be dangerous

- **Pearl**

Mortality is related to the underlying malignancy rather than the presence of superior vena caval obstruction.

Reference

Markman M: Diagnosis and management of superior vena cava syndrome. Cleve Clin J Med 1999;66:59. [PMID: 9926632]

Tumor Lysis Syndrome

- **Essentials of Diagnosis**
  - Recent administration of chemotherapy for treatment of a rapidly proliferating malignancy with massive destruction of neoplastic cells; described in Burkitt lymphoma and some leukemias without precipitating chemotherapy
  - Lysis of cells leads to hyperkalemia, hyperphosphatemia, hyperuricemia
  - Hyperphosphatemia associated with hypocalcemia
  - Hyperuricemia can cause uric acid nephropathy, renal failure
  - Symptoms related to metabolic and electrolyte changes
  - Complications: electrocardiographic changes, cardiac arrhythmias, tetany, convulsions, oliguria, muscle cramps, lethargy

- **Differential Diagnosis**
  - Burkitt lymphoma
  - Acute lymphocytic leukemia
  - Chronic lymphocytic leukemia
  - Solid tumors
  - Spontaneous necrosis of malignancies

- **Treatment**
  - Aggressive volume resuscitation
  - Prevention of hyperuricemia with allopurinol before administration of chemotherapy
  - Appropriate treatment for hyperkalemia and hyperphosphatemia
  - Alkalinization of urine (pH 7.0–7.5) while serum uric acid levels are elevated
  - Hemodialysis for life-threatening electrolyte abnormalities and renal failure

- **Pearl**

High leukocyte and platelet counts may cause pseudohyperkalemia due to lysis of these cells after blood collection. No electrocardiographic abnormalities will be seen, and plasma instead of serum potassium should be followed.

Reference

Gobel BH: Management of tumor lysis syndrome: prevention and treatment. Semin Oncol Nurs 2002;18:12. [PMID: 12184047]

20

Pregnancy

Acute Fatty Liver of Pregnancy

- **Essentials of Diagnosis**
  - Hepatic dysfunction associated with liver biopsy demonstrating microvesicular fatty infiltration of hepatocytes
  - Nausea, vomiting, varying degrees of epigastric and right upper quadrant pain, anorexia, malaise
  - Most commonly occurs in third trimester and immediate post-partum period
  - Aspartate aminotransferase (AST) and alanine aminotransferase (ALT) usually <1000 IU/L; alkaline phosphatase and bilirubin increase, albumin decreases, WBC elevated, coagulopathy consistent with disseminated intravascular coagulopathy (DIC), hypoglycemia
  - Increased incidence in first pregnancies, twin gestations
  - Complications: fulminant hepatic failure, hypoglycemia, consumptive coagulopathy, renal failure, cerebral edema, pancreatitis, spontaneous labor, fetal demise

- **Differential Diagnosis**
  - Preeclampsia/eclampsia
  - Budd-Chiari syndrome
  - Cholestasis of pregnancy
  - HELLP syndrome (hemolysis, elevated liver enzymes, low platelets)
  - Fulminant hepatic failure secondary to medications
  - Acute hepatic rupture
  - Viral hepatitis

- **Treatment**
  - Continuous fetal monitoring until delivery
  - Maintain patent airway if mental obtundation present; normalize intravascular volume status; correct electrolyte disturbances; dextrose infusions to support hypoglycemia; correct hematologic and coagulation abnormalities
  - Delivery should be performed as soon as patient stabilized; delays can result in fetal demise from uteroplacental insufficiency or hypoglycemia; clinical improvement typically follows
  - Supportive measures: nutritional support to prevent hypoglycemia; consider lactulose or other ammonia reducing agents if encephalopathic; administer vitamin K if coagulopathic

- **Pearl**

AFLP can present with such nonspecific findings as nausea, vomiting, and right upper quadrant pain that the diagnosis can be overlooked with drastic consequences including fulminant hepatic failure if treatment is delayed.

Reference

Sandhu BS et al: Pregnancy and liver disease. Gastroenterol Clin North Am 2003;32:407. [PMID: 12635424]

Amniotic Fluid Embolism

- **Essentials of Diagnosis**
  - Dyspnea and hypotension followed by sudden cardiovascular collapse
  - Greatest risk during active labor; also reported after vaginal or Cesarean delivery, following termination of first or second trimester pregnancy
  - Coagulopathy, seizures, pulmonary edema, ARDS, fetal distress
  - Echocardiography reveals left ventricular dysfunction in addition to only mild to moderate pulmonary hypertension
  - Appears triggered by release of amniotic fluid and debris into maternal pulmonary circulation
  - Classic finding of fetal squamous cells in maternal pulmonary circulation at autopsy; difficult to distinguish maternal from fetal origin of cells if drawn from central catheter premortem
  - High maternal mortality rate with all deaths occurring within 5 hours of presentation; only 15% of survivors neurologically intact

- **Differential Diagnosis**
  - Pulmonary embolism
  - Acute myocardial infarction
  - Placental rupture
  - Adverse reaction to anesthetic agents
  - Septic shock
  - Peripartum cardiomyopathy
  - Anaphylaxis

- **Treatment**
  - Maintain oxygenation with mechanical ventilation and application of positive end-expiratory pressure (PEEP); circulatory support with volume and vasopressors; consider inotropic agents to improve myocardial function; pulmonary artery catheter may be helpful in directing therapy; correction of coagulopathy
  - Consider prompt delivery of fetus if maternal cardiopulmonary arrest as this may improve likelihood of success of resuscitation

- **Pearl**

Amniotic fluid embolism should be suspected in the pregnant or postpartum woman who develops sudden unexpected cardiovascular collapse.

Reference

Davies S: Amniotic fluid embolus: a review of the literature. Can J Anaesth 2001;48:88. [PMID: 11212056]

Asthma in Pregnancy

- **Essentials of Diagnosis**
  - Dyspnea, chest tightness, wheezing, cough
  - Accessory muscle use, wheezing, prolonged expiratory phase, tachypnea, tachycardia
  - Interpret arterial blood gases in light of physiologic changes associated with pregnancy in which $Paco_2$ is reduced; development of "hypercapnia" may be subtle sign of impending respiratory failure
  - Increased risk of complications if asthma history reveals hospitalizations, intubations, prolonged steroid use, pneumothorax
  - Adverse effects on pregnancy when maternal hypoxemia affects oxygenation of fetus: premature labor, low birth weights, increased risk of fetal death

- **Differential Diagnosis**
  - Congestive heart failure
  - Pneumothorax
  - Pulmonary embolism
  - Dyspnea due to physiologic and mechanical changes of pregnancy

- **Treatment**
  - Spirometry useful for assessing severity and following response to therapy
  - Beta-agonists should be titrated to clinical response
  - Oral corticosteroids well tolerated and should be considered for use in exacerbations; inhaled corticosteroids may be helpful in maintaining asthma control
  - Supplemental oxygen to maintain $Pao_2 > 85$ mm Hg to ensure adequate fetal oxygenation
  - If infectious contribution suspected, avoid certain antibiotics in pregnancy: sulfonamides, erythromycin estolate, tetracycline, chloramphenicol, quinolones
  - Consider mechanical ventilation if severe hypoxemia, mental status changes, respiratory acidosis, cardiac arrhythmias, myocardial ischemia

- **Pearl**

A $Paco_2$ greater than 35 mm Hg in a pregnant woman may be a sign of impending respiratory failure during a severe asthma exacerbation as the normal range of $Paco_2$ in pregnancy is 28 to 32 mm Hg.

Reference

Graves CR: Acute pulmonary complications during pregnancy. Clin Obstet Gynecol 2002;45:369. [PMID: 12048396]

Preeclampsia and Eclampsia

- **Essentials of Diagnosis**
  - Preeclampsia classically defined as clinical triad of hypertension, proteinuria, edema; because of frequency of edema in pregnancy, edema has been omitted from diagnostic criterion
  - Severe preeclampsia characterized by additional features: blood pressure >160/110, more proteinuria, elevated creatinine, pulmonary edema, oliguria, hemolytic anemia, liver dysfunction, fetal growth restriction
  - Eclampsia defined by addition of seizures without known cause
  - May be complicated by HELLP syndrome
  - Occurs in previously normotensive patients or with preexisting chronic hypertension after 20 weeks gestation; develops earlier with multiple fetuses, hydatiform mole

- **Differential Diagnosis**
  - Chronic essential hypertension
  - Gestational hypertension
  - Acute fatty liver of pregnancy
  - Chronic renal disease

- **Treatment**
  - Delivery of fetus definitive treatment; delays while administering antihypertensive therapy remains controversial
  - Seizure prophylaxis and control with magnesium sulfate from day of diagnosis until delivery; therapeutic goal range 4.8–8.4 mg/dL
  - Hypertension control if blood pressure >180/110 with agents including hydralazine and labetalol; in severe cases nitroprusside may be used for limited time due to potential fetal cyanide poisoning
  - Pulmonary artery catheter monitoring if oliguria unresponsive to fluids, pulmonary edema unresponsive to diuretics and positional changes, or severe hypertension unresponsive to conventional therapy

- **Pearl**

The only known definitive treatment for preeclampsia-eclampsia syndrome is delivery of the fetus.

Reference

Roberts JM et al: Summary of the NHLBI working group on research on hypertension during pregnancy. Hypertension 2003;41;437. [PMID: 12623940]

Pulmonary Edema in Pregnancy

- **Essentials of Diagnosis**
  - Dyspnea, cough, chest discomfort, frothy sputum, hypoxemia
  - Bilateral rales; other signs of overt heart failure may be absent
  - Chest radiograph with interstitial or alveolar infiltrates and perihilar congestion; unilateral edema possible
  - Can occur without known predisposing conditions and typically presents at time of delivery
  - Associated conditions: hypertension; undiagnosed heart conditions, especially mitral stenosis; tocolytic agents; fluid overload; peripartum cardiomyopathy
  - Proposed mechanisms: fluid overload due to increased extracellular volume during pregnancy; fluid administration during labor; increased capillary permeability; decreased plasma oncotic pressure
  - Echocardiography helpful in evaluating valvular heart disease or cardiomyopathy

- **Differential Diagnosis**
  - Pulmonary embolism
  - Asthma
  - Peripartum cardiomyopathy
  - Amniotic fluid embolism
  - Myocardial ischemia

- **Treatment**
  - Majority improve dramatically within 24 hours of treatment
  - Discontinue tocolytic agents
  - Intravenous loop diuretics
  - Supplemental oxygen to maintain adequate saturations
  - Antibiotics should be administered if infection suspected
  - Continuous fetal heart monitoring until normal maternal pulmonary function restored and hypoxemia has resolved; if fetus affected, late decelerations and loss of heart rate variability may be noted
  - If slow in resolving, suspect structural cardiac abnormalities; echocardiography and pulmonary artery catheter may be helpful in guiding therapy in these settings

- **Pearl**

The physiologic adaptations to pregnancy, including increased cardiac output, decreased systemic vascular resistance, and decreased colloid oncotic pressure, predispose to the development of pulmonary edema.

Reference

Siscione AC et al: Acute pulmonary edema in pregnancy. Obstet Gynecol 2003;101:511. [PMID: 12636955]

Pyelonephritis in Pregnancy

- ■ Essentials of Diagnosis
  - • Flank pain (right side > left), fever, rigors, chills
  - • May complain of lower urinary tract symptoms including dysuria, frequency
  - • Ominous signs: hypotension, tachypnea, marked tachycardia, high fever
  - • Pyuria nearly always present; red blood cells and casts frequently found; urine cultures should be obtained to confirm diagnosis and evaluate for antibiotic resistance
  - • *E coli* most frequent organism identified
  - • Risk of recurrence increases after first episode
  - • Adverse effects: uterine contractions and premature birth
  - • Pathogenesis related to ureteral relaxation from increased progesterone levels leading to urinary stasis; bacteria from lower genitourinary tract ascend to kidneys

- ■ Differential Diagnosis
  - • Intra-amniotic infection
  - • Appendicitis
  - • Renal stones
  - • Cholecystitis

- ■ Treatment
  - • Initially treat as inpatient because of greater incidence of severe complications including septic shock and ARDS
  - • Antibiotics mainstay of treatment with agents chosen empirically to cover major community acquired urinary pathogens
  - • Supportive care: volume resuscitation; aggressive antipyretics and cooling blankets to prevent premature uterine contractures and fetal neurologic harm from prolonged exposure to febrile state
  - • Continuous fetal heart monitoring for all pregnancies beyond 22 weeks gestation
  - • Some advocate prophylactic antibiotics throughout pregnancy after first episode; others suggest monitoring with serial urine cultures

- ■ Pearl
Bacteriuria in pregnancy predisposes women to the development of acute pyelonephritis which can be complicated by preterm labor.

Reference
Gilstrap LC III et al: Urinary tract infections during pregnancy. Obstet Gynecol Clin North Am 2001;28:581. [PMID: 11512502]

Septic Abortion

- **Essentials of Diagnosis**
  - Sepsis syndrome following recent spontaneous or induced pregnancy termination
  - Crampy pelvic pain with serosanguineous or purulent vaginal discharge occurring within 7 days of recent pregnancy termination or other intrauterine instrumentation
  - Hematuria and shock can develop rapidly
  - Abdominal and pelvic exam with tenderness and possible peritoneal signs; dilated cervix, lacerations, products of conception, bleeding, discharge
  - Blood, urine, and cervical specimens should be obtained for culture
  - Polymicrobial infection with aerobic and anaerobic organisms; *Clostridium* species important pathogens and suggested by large gram-positive rods on Gram stain
  - Abdominal radiographs helpful in diagnosis of uterine or bowel perforation; gas in myometrium noted on radiographs consistent with clostridial infection and carries grave prognosis; ultrasound to assess for presence of retained products of conception or detecting possible pelvic abscesses
  - Likelihood of complications increases with later abortions or with dilation and evacuation procedures

- **Differential Diagnosis**
  - Perforated viscus
  - Septic shock from prolonged rupture of membranes
  - Puerperal sepsis

- **Treatment**
  - Prompt broad-spectrum antibiotics followed by planned uterine evacuation procedure
  - Hysterectomy may be life saving if clostridial infection suspected by discolored dusky uterus with myonecrosis or crepitation
  - Supportive management of accompanying complications including ARDS, hypotension, anemia, shock

- **Pearl**

Septic abortion is usually a polymicrobial infection with aerobic and anaerobic bacteria including sexually transmitted pathogens and Clostridial species.

Reference

Tamussino K: Postoperative infection. Clin Obstet Gynecol 2002;45:562. (PMID: 12048413)

Index